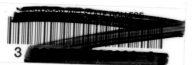

Eat Well
&
Keep Moving

An Interdisciplinary Curriculum for Teaching Upper Elementary School Nutrition and Physical Activity

Lilian W. Y. Cheung, DSc, RD
Harvard School of Public Health

Steven L. Gortmaker, PhD
Harvard School of Public Health

Hank Dart, MS
Health Communication Consultant

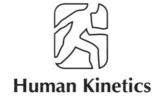

Human Kinetics

Library of Congress Cataloging-in-Publication Data

Cheung, Lilian W. Y., 1951-
    Eat well and keep moving : an interdisciplinary curriculum for teaching upper
elementary school nutrition and physical activity / Lilian W.Y. Cheung, Steven L.
Gortmaker, Hank Dart.
        p. cm.
    Includes bibliographical references.
    ISBN 0-7360-3096-4
        1. Nutrition--Study and teaching (Elementary) 2. Exercise--Study and teaching
(Elementary) I. Gortmaker, Steven Lawrence, 1949- II. Dart, Hank, 1967- III. Title.

TX364 .C44 2000
372.3'7--dc21

                                                                                00-040767

ISBN: 0-7360-3096-4

Micro-units contributed by Planet Health.

Acquisitions Editor: Scott Wikgren; **Developmental Editor:** Amy N. Pickering; **Assistant Editors:** Derek Campbell, Sandra Merz-Bott; **Copyeditor:** Brian Mustain; **Proofreader:** Pam Johnson; **Permission Manager:** Courtney Astle; **Graphic Designer:** Nancy Rasmus; **Graphic Artist:** Denise Lowry; **Cover Designer:** Jack W. Davis; **Photographer (interior):** Tom Roberts; **Illustrator:** Tom Roberts, Sharon Smith, Denise Lowry; **Printer:** Versa Press

Printed in the United States of America   10   9   8   7   6   5   4   3   2   1

Human Kinetics
Web site: www.humankinetics.com

United States: Human Kinetics, P.O. Box 5076, Champaign, IL 61825-5076
800-747-4457
e-mail: humank@hkusa.com

Canada: Human Kinetics, 475 Devonshire Road Unit 100, Windsor, ON N8Y 2L5
800-465-7301 (in Canada only)
e-mail: hkcan@mnsi.net

Europe: Human Kinetics, P.O. Box IW14, Leeds LS16 6TR, United Kingdom
+44 (0) 113 278 1708
e-mail: humank@hkeurope.com

Australia: Human Kinetics, 57A Price Avenue, Lower Mitcham, South Australia 5062
08 8277 1555
e-mail: liahka@senet.com.au

New Zealand: Human Kinetics, P.O. Box 105-231, Auckland Central
09-523-3462
e-mail: hkp@ihug.co.nz

To all children, educators,
and school food service personnel

Contents

Preface

Eat Well & *Keep Moving* is a school-based program that equips children with the knowledge, skills, and supportive environment they need to lead more healthful lives by choosing nutritious diets and being physically active. Research shows that a good diet and adequate physical activity can significantly reduce the risks of obesity and chronic diseases such as heart disease, high blood pressure, and diabetes, which can begin early in childhood. However, many children are not eating the food and getting the exercise they need to combat these chronic diseases and promote lifelong good health. Especially disconcerting is that as children age and move into adolescence and then adulthood, they become progressively less active and choose less-healthy diets. This makes it even more important for children to develop healthful habits early in life so that these practices can be sustained into adulthood.

The Eat Well & *Keep Moving* program was launched to provide teachers and school staff with the tools that students need to lead healthier lives. Initially designed as a joint research project between the Harvard School of Public Health and Baltimore City Public Schools, Eat Well & *Keep Moving* has evolved into a comprehensive program that can be introduced in other school systems throughout the country, including urban sites.

Unlike traditional health curricula, Eat Well & *Keep Moving* is a multifaceted program encompassing all aspects of the learning environment—from the classroom, the cafeteria, and the gymnasium to school hallways, the home, and even community centers. This comprehensive approach, as recommended by the Centers for Disease Control and Prevention, helps reinforce important messages about nutrition and physical activity, and it increases the chance that students will eat well and keep moving throughout their lives.

Numerous curricula exist that address either nutrition or physical activity independently, yet few address nutrition and physical activity simultaneously. This program is a significant addition to elementary school curricula because this is not only among the first to address both nutrition *and* physical activity, but it is also among the first to address children's physical inactivity, namely television viewing and computer game playing. Its six interlinked components—classroom education, physical education, school-wide promotional campaigns, food services, staff wellness, and parent involvement—work together to create a supportive learning environment that promotes the learning of lifelong good habits. But Eat Well & *Keep Moving* does not just work well for students. That it uses existing school resources, fits within most school curricula, contains camera-ready teaching materials, and is inexpensive to implement makes it easy for teachers and schools to adopt as well. Feedback from the teachers who have taught the curriculum has been exceptionally positive.

Eat Well & *Keep Moving* is a program you can make as large or as focused as you would like. Choose the approach that works best for you. Focusing solely on the classroom portion of the program will provide students with an excellent set of knowledge and skills that they can apply throughout life. The program is at its strongest, though, when it includes the entire school community: other teachers (classroom and physical education), food service staff, and parents or guardians. The power of the Eat Well & *Keep Moving* messages is enhanced even further when students are exposed to them in other classes, experience them in the cafeteria and school hallways, and put them into practice at home with their parents or guardians.

The Eat Well & *Keep Moving* book and accompanying CD-ROM provide all the information you need to implement the program, whether introducing it into a single classroom or expanding it to an entire school community or school system. The CD-ROM allows you to customize the content of the program according to your school and student population profile. For example, schools can tailor the foods, language, and customs of the lesson plans and activities to their student population.

Eat Well & *Keep Moving* Program Components

Parts I and II of the Eat Well & *Keep Moving* book contain the interdisciplinary fourth- and fifth-grade classroom lessons that provide students with the in-depth exposure to the program's nutrition and physical activity themes. Unique to these lessons, students learn about nutrition and physical activity while actually being physically active in the classroom. This is especially valuable in schools where physical education is limited or not available.

Part III, promotions for the classroom, offers students and teachers fun and engaging ways to put the themes of the program into practice. These promotions include walking clubs, the Get 3-at-School & 5-A-Day promotion, the *Freeze My TV* contest, and the Pyramid Power Game.

Parts IV, V, VI, and VII contain the physical education lessons, the FitChecks, the FitCheck physical education micro-units, and the additional physical education micro-units. The physical education lessons offer students more traditional physical education activities, many of which also integrate nutrition topics. Students learn as they move and, by doing so, begin to appreciate the importance of both eating well and being physically active. The FitCheck is a tool for self-assessment of activity and inactivity. Teachers and students are taught how to use this tool in order to evaluate how students are progressing. The FitCheck physical education micro-units were designed to be used with the FitCheck materials to teach students about a variety of topics in physical activity. Likewise, the additional physical education micro-units are five-minute-long "brief lessons" that cover a wide range of physical activity topics.

You will notice that both the FitCheck micro-units and the additional micro-units have been formatted differently than the rest of the book. These units use many bulleted lists to provide you with an easy outline to follow while you are delivering the lessons to your students. Likewise, you will notice text boxes within the micro-units. These text boxes contain additional information that you can share with your students to help them learn even more about the topic at hand.

The appendix provides references on stretches and strength exercises that will be used throughout the book, and it houses the Eat Well & *Keep Moving* cards. These cards offer a quick and fun way for students to synthesize and put into practice the nutrition and physical activity information they learn through the lessons and other promotions.

The Eat Well & *Keep Moving* CD-ROM provides in-depth implementation manuals and supporting materials for each part of the program as well as information for running workshops to train fellow teachers, food service staff, and community members about nutrition and physical education. It also contains the classroom and physical education lessons contained in this book so that you can personalize the worksheets and other reproducibles with your own school logos.

Even more important than the scope of your school's approach to implementing the Eat Well & *Keep Moving* program is the fact that you are teaching your students how important it is to Eat Well & *Keep Moving*. It will not only help them be healthier, happier students right now, but it will also give them the knowledge and skills they need for lifelong good health.

Acknowledgments

The Eat Well & *Keep Moving* program was developed over a five-year period by a team headed by Lilian Cheung and Steven Gortmaker. The ideas for the programs evolved among the faculty at the Harvard School of Public Health after the 1991 Harvard Conference on Nutrition and Physical Activity for Youth, co-chaired by Lilian Cheung and Julius Richmond. In 1993, the program began in earnest with support from Christy and John Walton of the Walton Family Foundation. Christy Walton had long been concerned about the state of children's nutrition and the role of public schools. She introduced Lilian Cheung and her colleagues to the Baltimore City Public Schools, where the pilot program for Eat Well & *Keep Moving* started in 1993. Research documenting the effectiveness of Eat Well & *Keep Moving* was published in 1999 (Gortmaker et al. 1999). The program was such a resounding success that the Baltimore City Department of Education has now made it available to all public elementary schools in Baltimore.

Eat Well & *Keep Moving* was the result of a strong collaboration among faculty members from the Departments of Nutrition, Health and Social Behavior, Maternal and Child Health, Epidemiology, and Biostatistics at the Harvard School of Public Health. The team of co-investigators included Lilian Cheung, Steven Gortmaker, Karen Peterson, Graham Colditz, and Nan Laird. Eat Well & *Keep Moving* owes its success to *many, many* dedicated individuals, spanning a wide range of expertise including educators, academic researchers, nutritionists, food service specialists, and physical education teachers. The authors wish to thank those listed in the following paragraphs for their dedication, hard work, and perseverance. Eat Well & *Keep Moving* would never have become a reality without them.

Our sincerest thanks to our Harvard team, including Ginny Chomitz for her leadership role early on and for overseeing process evaluation; Jay Hammond Cradle, our strategic liaison between Harvard and Baltimore who truly made it possible for the program to be a success; Marianne Lee for her skillful project management; Wendy Fraser, Julie Fredericksen, and Ronita Wisniewski for coordinating the project as well as playing key roles in materials development; Karen Peterson for her global vision of public health nutrition and the importance of intervention studies; Graham Colditz and Alison Field for their insights and forthright advice; Nan Laird for her guidance in statistical methods; and Kevin Morris, Shari Sprong, Shirley Hung, Kelley Wells, Darlene Ratliff, and Teresa Fung for their input into the manuals. We owe special thanks to Barbara Lind for leading retreats that inspired us all and to Jon Chomitz for his artistic inputs in the photographic essay and the design of the Eat Well & *Keep Moving* logo. We thank Helen Klipp for helping us pull together the Eat Well & *Keep Moving* grant.

Special thanks to authors of the Planet Health Micro-Units (Carter et al. 2000), Jill Carter, Jean Wiecha, Karen Peterson, and Steven Gortmaker, for adapting 11 units for use with Eat Well & *Keep Moving*. We thank Karen Morse for her contribution of ideas to the micro-units.

We are grateful to the support of Harvey Fineberg, Harvard University provost, and Barry Bloom, dean of the Harvard School of Public Health, for endorsing Eat Well & *Keep Moving*. We thank Walter Willett, chair of the department of nutrition, for his wise counsel and his unwavering support. We appreciate too the efforts of John Lichten at the Harvard School of Public Health and Stewart Springfield at the Walton Family Foundation for their skillful assistance in the contract management, and Eleanor Livingston for her administrative support.

We owe a great debt of gratitude to our other colleagues in Baltimore; special thanks to Reba Bullock and Edith Fulmore of the Department of Curriculum and Instruction for working with us in development of the classroom lessons and teacher trainings, as well as assistance from their colleagues Andrea Boyer, April Lewis, and Brenda Holmes. Vivian Brake for playing a leading role in the food service programs, Jan Desper Maybin for her staff wellness work, Alanna Taylor for parental involvement components, and Ruth Bushnell for her innovative work in creating classroom-based physical activity lesson plans. Special thanks go to Former Superintendent Walter Amprey; Matthew Riley of the Baltimore City Department of Education; Leonard Smackum, director of the Department of Food and Nutrition Services, and his colleagues Joann Bell, Shirley Kane, and Kathleen Wilson.

Eat Well & *Keep Moving* would never have left the drawing board without the dedication of the principals from the collaborating schools. They are truly the unsung heroines who continue to inspire and nurture their students. Thank you for their honest feedback and guidance. Specifically, we want to recognize Doris Graham of Dr. Rayner Browne Elementary School; Rosemunde Smith and Flora Johnson of Mary E. Rodman Elementary School; Shirley Johnson of Edgewood Elementary School; Ann Moore of Sarah M. Roach Elementary School; Janice Noranbrock of Mildred Monroe Elementary School; and Julia Winder of Graceland Park-O'Donnell Heights. In addition, we would like to thank the principals from participating schools: Bernice Welcher of City Springs Elementary School; Barbara Hill and Betty Ross of George Street Elementary School; Iris Harris of Collington Square Elementary School; Addie Johnson of Robert W. Coleman Elementary School; Mayess Craig of Walter P. Carter Elementary School; Dale Parker-Brown and Patricia Dennis of Montebello Elementary School; Margaret Wicks and Jean Tien of Holabird Elementary School; and Elizabeth L. Turner of Tench Tilghman Elementary School.

We would like to thank all lead teachers and teachers who assisted in the training and evaluation of the program: Verbena Redmond of Dr. Rayner Browne Elementary School; Sandra Watt of Edgewood Elementary School; Myra Smith of Graceland Park-O'Donnell Heights; Marian J. McCrea of Mary E. Rodman Elementary School; Cecelia Cooper of Mildred Monroe Elementary School; and Dorothy M. Simpson of Sarah M. Roach Elementary School. We especially appreciate the efforts of the fourth- and fifth-grade teachers in Baltimore elementary schools who taught the lessons and gave us valuable feedback. Moreover, we express our gratitude to all food service staff, students, parent liaisons, and parents in participating schools.

We acknowledge with thanks the assistance provided by volunteer organizations in Baltimore: Sandra Esslinger and Connie Stewart of American Cancer Society; Barbara Brisco, Patricia Finch, Amanda Self, and Gwendolyn Jackson of Maryland Cooperative Extension Services; Tracy Newsom, Brenda Schwab, and Theresa Lance of Maryland Food Committee; Tammy Jo Walker and Sandy Stewart of National Black Women's Health Project; and Susan Jackson-Speed of Operation Frontline.

Special thanks are due to Abt Associates, especially Mary Kay Fox for her leadership and competence in managing data collection, and Mary Jo Cutler for her input in food service and training. Thanks to Lorelei DiSogra and Dole Food Company for their generous gifts of promotional materials for our Get 3-at-School & 5-A-Day promotion. We thank Scott Wikgren, Amy Pickering, and their talented editorial staff at Human Kinetics, Inc. for their help in making Eat Well & *Keep Moving* available nationally and internationally.

We are very grateful for the guidance of a distinguished advisory board: William Dietz (chair), Cheryl Achterberg, Dorothy Caldwell, Janet Collins, Dale Conoscenti, Tony Earls, John Foreyt, David Herzog, Nancy Harmon Jenkins, Sue Kimm, Katherine Merseth, Julius Richmond, Alex Roche, James Sallis, Cassandra Simmons, and Walter Willett. We thank the United States Department of Agriculture for recognizing the excellence of this program in granting Eat Well & *Keep Moving* a Promising Practice award in 1997.

We express our gratitude to the Walton Family Foundation for the generous funding that brought this project to life, and in particular we thank John and Christy Walton for years of supporting and championing this project. Finally, we thank all the children who participated in Eat Well & *Keep Moving*. Their critiques gave us invaluable insights toward developing a successful program. They continue to inspire us, and we wish them a healthy and bright future.

Lilian Cheung
Steven Gortmaker
Hank Dart
May 2000

Carter J, Wiecha J, Peterson KE, Gortmaker SL. *Planet Health.* Human Kinetics Press, 2000.

Gortmaker SL, Cheung LWY, Peterson KE, Chomitz G, Cradle JH, Dart H, Fox MK, Bullock RB, Sobol AM, Colditz G, Field A, Laird N. Impact of a school-based interdisciplinary intervention on diet and physical activity among urban primary school children: Eat Well and *Keep Moving*. Archives of Pediatrics and Adolescent Medicine. 1999;153:975-83.

Introduction

The Eat Well & *Keep Moving* book is divided into two main sections: section 1, which contains the classroom lessons and promotions, and section 2, which contains the physical education lessons and micro-units. In addition, you can use the Eat Well & *Keep Moving* CD-ROM to expand the program beyond your classroom to food services, other teachers, and students' homes.

Section 1

The classroom component of Eat Well & *Keep Moving* (parts I–III) combines nutrition and physical activity lessons, discussion cards (Eat Well cards and Keep Moving cards), and promotional activities to create a reinforcing and supportive learning environment for students.

The lessons on nutrition and physical activity are the most prominent feature of the classroom component. The 12 multidisciplinary lessons for fourth and fifth grades provide students the knowledge and skills they need to choose healthful eating patterns and be physically active. Developed with elementary school teachers, these lessons

- are meant to be integrated into core subject areas;
- follow a format familiar to educators;
- meet educational standards;
- require minimal teacher training; and
- are simple, clear, and easy to use.

Parts I and II: Classroom Lessons on Nutrition and Physical Activity

The classroom lessons on nutrition and physical activity comprise the cornerstone of Eat Well & *Keep Moving*. The fourth-grade (part I) and fifth-grade (part II) lessons use multidisciplinary teaching and unique approaches to equip students with the knowledge and lifelong skills they need to choose a nutritious diet and be physically active.

Designed to fit easily into a school's curriculum, the lessons address a wide range of learning outcomes and can be taught across numerous subject matter areas (such as math, language arts, social studies, and visual arts). See the table on the next page for a detailed list of learning outcomes/competencies addressed by the classroom lessons. Depending on the school, the lessons can either be taught as part of the regular core subjects or health education.

Messages of the Lessons

The Eat Well & *Keep Moving* classroom lessons focus on five simple messages. Students should do the following:

- Eat at least five servings of fruits and vegetables a day
- Eat less fat (especially saturated and *trans* fat)
- Eat a nutritious breakfast every morning
- Be more physically active
- Be less physically inactive (specifically, they should watch less television)

Eat Well & *Keep Moving* Education Components

Classroom Activity	#	Description
Parts I and II—Classroom Lessons		
Part I—Grade 4	12	Classroom lessons on the topics of wellness, the Food Guide Pyramid, 5-A-Day (fruits and vegetables), snacking, limiting television, and the safe workout
Part II—Grade 5	12	Classroom lessons on the topics of wellness, the Food Guide Pyramid, 5-A-Day (fruits and vegetables), snacking, limiting television, and the safe workout
Part III—Promotional Activities		
Walking clubs	1	Yearlong class-walking clubs
Freeze My TV	1	Weeklong activity focusing on limiting time students spend watching television
Get 3-at-School & 5-A-Day	1	Weeklong activity focusing in getting 3 serving of fruits and vegetables while at school and totaling 5 servings for the entire day
Pyramid Power	1	A repeating game that helps teach and reinforce the messages of the Food Guide Pyramid
Eat Well cards	18	Brief discussions focusing primarily on healthful selections in the cafeteria
Keep Moving cards	2	Brief discussion of physical activity topics addressed in the classroom and physical education lessons
Part IV, V, VI, VII—Physical Education Activities		
Grade 4/5 lessons	5	Physical education lessons following the safe workout format while also addressing nutrition issues
Grade 4/5 micro-units	9	Five-minute activities teaching a variety of nutrition and physical education topics

Through lessons on overall health, the Food Guide Pyramid, and safe physical workouts, students learn why these messages are important and are given the knowledge and skills to put them into practice.

Lesson Format

The Eat Well & *Keep Moving* lessons are very clear and easy to use. Each lesson is described step by step, and background information is provided for each teacher's use at the beginning of each lesson. An overhead projector and copies made from the worksheet masters are two of the few materials needed that are not included with the lessons.

The lessons are designed to be integrated into various core subjects and disciplines (e.g., language arts, math, science, health, social studies, and art). This not only allows the lesson to fit more easily into the class schedule, but it also spreads the program's message even further across all facets of the students' school day.

Physical Activity Lessons for the Classroom

One of the many unique aspects of the Eat Well & *Keep Moving* classroom lessons is that a number of the lessons teach nutrition and physical activity issues while students are actually moving in the classroom. This approach reinforces the importance of eating a nutritious diet and being physically active. Addressing both issues simultaneously, as certain lessons do, helps convey this link to students. Second, getting students moving in the classroom can supplement a school's physical education program.

The basic structure of the physical activity classroom lessons is based on a five-part framework called "the safe workout." Essentially, the safe workout teaches students the safe way to be physically active.

Each physical activity lesson actually leads students through the five steps:

1. Warm-up
2. Stretch
3. Fitness activity—an active game that involves a nutrition concept
4. Cool-down
5. Cool-down stretch

After the cool-down stretch, students then gather in the "Stay Healthy Corner" and review what they learned during the lesson.

These safe workout lessons were designed to be used in a variety of settings. While they work best in an area with a fair amount of open space (such as a gymnasium and cafeteria), they have also been successfully taught in the classroom itself with urban schools having class sizes of up to 30 students a class (usually with a slight rearranging of furniture).

To get a large, varied collection of food pictures to use in the physical activity lessons (as well as in some of the nutrition lessons and physical education lessons), teachers can ask students to bring in a number of pictures (from magazines, etc.) or empty packages in the weeks before the lessons are going to be taught. It is probably never too early to begin such a collection. Sets of approximately 100 food pictures may also be purchased from the National Dairy Council for around $25. Contact the National Dairy Council at 1-800-426-8271.

Part III: Classroom Promotions and the Eat Well Cards and Keep Moving Cards

The Eat Well & *Keep Moving* program includes four classroom promotions that build upon the classroom lessons and provide students the opportunity to put their nutrition and physical activity knowledge into practice over an extended period of time.

Class-Walking Clubs

The class-walking clubs can run throughout the school year and arise directly from the Fitness Walking lessons. Classes are encouraged to chart walking routes around their school and to go on walks with their teacher at least once a week. To add interest to the club, classes are encouraged to "walk" across a part of the world. Each time they walk they can accrue a certain number of miles (for example, every 5 minutes equals 100 miles) and mark their progress on a map.

Freeze My TV

Freeze My TV is an activity where students keep track of and try to limit the amount of television they watch for an entire week. The Freeze My TV activity ties directly to fourth-grade lesson 8 and fifth-grade lesson 19. In addition to keeping track of the time they spend watching television, students also complete graphing activities, answer questions based on their graphs, and make entries each day in the *Freeze My TV Journal*.

Watching television and playing video games are the main contributors to a sedentary lifestyle. Getting students to limit the amount of television they watch frees up more time for them to spend being physically active (such as riding their bikes or dancing) or working on more worthwhile projects (such as drawing or reading). One idea for supplementing Freeze My TV with art is having students create colorful posters with catchy slogans to display these alternatives to watching television.

Get 3-at-School & 5-A-Day

Students put their knowledge of healthful eating into practice in this weeklong activity by trying to consume at least three servings of fruits and vegetables while at school. Each student tracks his or her at-school fruit and vegetable consumption on a large class graph. In addition to getting three servings of fruits and vegetables while at school, students are also encouraged to get a total of five servings for the entire day. To help reach this goal, students are encouraged to take materials home that reinforce the 5-A-Day message (such as the *Fun with Fruits and Vegetables Cookbook* and *5 A Day Tracking Chart*, which are both available from Dole Foods for free).

Using Eat Well cards (described below) during the Get 3-at-School & 5-A-Day activity can further motivate students to eat their fruits and vegetables. These cards, many of which address fruits and vegetables, can be briefly discussed with students just before lunch during the week of the Get 3-at-School & 5-A-Day activity.

Pyramid Power Game

The Pyramid Power game turns the messages of the Food Guide Pyramid into a fun and edifying board game. Played in groups or as an entire class, the Pyramid Power game can serve as a daily review of the classroom and physical education lessons, as well as a refresher of the Eat Well & *Keep Moving* messages throughout the school year. The game consists of a set of question cards and a Food Guide Pyramid board, which depicts the number of recommended servings for each food group. When students answer the nutrition-related questions on the cards correctly, they receive points that go toward filling in the recommended servings on the pyramid game board. The first student or group to fill in all the servings wins the game.

Eat Well Cards and Keep Moving Cards

Eat Well cards and Keep Moving cards reinforce key messages and serve as important links between the classroom and the food services and physical education components of the program. Each card is 5.5 × 8.5 inches and contains a mixture of text and graphics. The cards present intriguing information that is intended to pique the interest of students and that can be reviewed with students in as little as three minutes. Although brief, the Eat Well cards and Keep Moving cards play an important role in helping students synthesize and put into practice the nutrition and physical activity information they learn through the program's lessons and other promotions. These cards can also be reprinted in a school's parent newsletter, providing an important link between home and school.

Eat Well Cards

Eat Well cards reinforce the nutrition messages of the classroom lessons and excite students about healthful choices on the cafeteria lunch menus. With their direct relationship to the cafeteria, Eat Well cards are designed to play an integral part of the Get 3-at-School & 5-A-Day activity in the classroom as well as support Eat Well & *Keep Moving*–related food service promotions.

On the Eat Well & *Keep Moving* Promotional Days (described in detail in the Food Services manual on the CD-ROM), a healthful food dish is highlighted each week in both the cafeteria and classroom. The dish is promoted to students in the cafeteria through table tents and posters during the week. On the day it is prepared, teachers present the appropriate Eat Well card just before students go off to lunch. This dual promotion helps motivate students to try the healthful dish.

Eat Well cards also remind students to eat their fruits and vegetables during the Get 3-at-School & 5-A-Day promotion, during which teachers are encouraged to review with students the Eat Well cards that address fruits and vegetables and the 5-A-Day theme.

Ideas for using Eat Well cards in the classroom:

- Review cards with students just before lunch on an appropriate day.
- Quiz students about the information contained in the card.
- Post the Eat Well cards on a bulletin board.
- Have a group of students review a card and present the information to the entire class.
- Have the cafeteria manager present a card to the class and talk about how food is prepared in the cafeteria.

Keep Moving Cards

Keep Moving cards are similar to Eat Well cards, but they discuss physical activity issues rather than nutrition issues. Topics covered by Keep Moving cards include stretching, warming up, and physical activity recommendations. Like Eat Well cards, Keep Moving cards can be discussed with students to bolster the messages students receive through other means, in this case the physical education class.

Ideas for using Keep Moving cards in the classroom:

- Review cards with students just before physical education class.
- Quiz students about the information contained in the card.
- Post the Keep Moving cards on a bulletin board.
- Have the physical education teacher come to class to present a card to the students.
- Have a group of students review a card and present the information to the entire class.

Section 2

The Eat Well & *Keep Moving* program has five physical education lessons and nine micro-units that complement a school's existing physical education curriculum. These lessons and micro-units are designed to help students develop a lifetime habit of physical activity. The lessons and micro-units not only provide students with the skills for a safe workout but also emphasize the importance of combining good nutrition and physical activity—a concept taught throughout the program's classroom lessons.

Although similar in format to the physical activity classroom lessons, the physical education lessons and micro-units are intended to be taught by the school's physical education teacher.

Lesson Format

In addition to the step-by-step description of the activity, safety concerns are addressed, and, where appropriate, a line drawing is included.

The basic structure of the physical education lessons is based on the five-part framework of the safe workout, described in section 1, although step 3 now focuses on an endurance fitness activity.

If the endurance activity game laid out in the lessons is less vigorous than your students are used to, they can begin each endurance fitness activity with a jog/walk, based on this schedule:

Lessons 29 and 30: Begin with a 4-minute jog/fast walk.

Lessons 31 and 32: Begin with a 5-minute jog/fast walk.

Lesson 33: Begin with a 6-minute jog/fast walk.

Because each Eat Well & *Keep Moving* physical education lesson addresses a nutrition topic, the physical education teacher may want to think about beginning a collection of food pictures, packages, and labels. Students can help with this process by bringing in items from home. Having access to such a collection will help make the endurance fitness activities more engaging to students. Physical education teachers and classroom teachers may wish to pool their collections.

Physical educators, in addition to receiving copies of the physical education lessons, should also have access to and become familiar with the program's fourth- and fifth-grade classroom lessons. This will help teachers make direct links between physical education and the classroom. In addition, having access to the classroom lessons will also allow physical educators to be a resource for classroom teachers who may have questions about some of the physical activity issues discussed in the classroom modules.

Micro-Units

The nine micro-units are brief, five-minute-long "lessons" that cover a wide range of physical activity and nutrition topics. On days when no full-length Eat Well & *Keep Moving* physical education lesson is being taught, a micro-unit can be presented at the beginning of class.

CD-ROM

You can use the material on the Eat Well & *Keep Moving* CD-ROM to make nutrition and physical activity a school-wide and community-wide priority. The classroom activities and physical education lessons are powerful teaching tools in their own right, but when the Eat Well & *Keep Moving* messages are expanded to the wider school community—as suggested by the Centers for Disease Control and Promotion—their impact on students becomes even greater.

Food Services

Outside of physical education, there is no clearer tie-in to Eat Well & *Keep Moving* than with school food services. Every school day, students eat at least one meal at school, providing an excellent opportunity to reinforce the messages of Eat Well & *Keep Moving*. This can be as simple as getting a cafeteria menu in advance and integrating it into your lessons or as involved as working with the principal and food service manager of your school to make permanent healthful changes to the school breakfast and lunch menus.

The CD-ROM provides detailed information for food services managers interested in making healthful changes to their school menus, including recipes, preparation tips, promotional material, classroom tie-ins, and staff training guides. When implemented to its fullest, the food service component works very closely with the classroom component, as explained in the promotions section of the CD-ROM.

The linkage between the classroom component of Eat Well & *Keep Moving* and the food services component can be strengthened if teachers and the cafeteria manager have an open dialogue about promoting the messages of the program. Teachers could invite the food service manager to give presentations in the classroom (such as an Eat Well card), and the cafeteria manager could provide teachers regular updates on scheduled lunch menus and display various Eat Well cards periodically on the serving line, complementing the lunch items served.

Parent Involvement

Parent involvement in Eat Well & *Keep Moving* is one of the keys to greatly bolstering the program's effectiveness. Encourage parents and family members to become involved in activities that complement the program messages students learn in school. This reinforcement increases the probability that the dietary and lifestyle changes students make will become a regular part of family and daily life.

As a teacher, you can volunteer some of your time to organize parent activities around Eat Well & *Keep Moving* messages, or you can locate a parent volunteer or other teacher to spearhead such activities. The CD-ROM details different approaches to getting parents and family members involved in Eat Well & *Keep Moving*. As with all the other components of the program, your level of involvement can be as little or as great as you like. The separate components of Eat Well & *Keep Moving* stand alone very well but become even stronger when brought together.

When implemented to its full extent, the parent involvement takes a unique approach: identifying community-based health organizations to offer nutrition, physical activity, and wellness programs to parents. Additional Eat Well & *Keep Moving* parent activities include publishing nutrition and physical activity information in school newsletters and hosting program-related family activities, such as Parent Fun Nights, which allow families to see exactly what their children are learning through the Eat Well & *Keep Moving* program.

Through these Eat Well & *Keep Moving*–related activities, it is our hope that parents/guardians will become models for their children and encourage and support healthy eating practices and active lifestyles for the entire family.

Other CD-ROM material

In addition to food service and parent involvement material, the CD-ROM also provides:

- Nutrition, physical activity, and wellness workshops for teachers;
- The complete fourth- and fifth-grade classroom and physical education lessons; and
- Information for school administrators interested in Eat Well & *Keep Moving*.

Putting It All Together

All the components of the Eat Well & *Keep Moving* program complement each other. Although each component can be used independently, the power of Eat Well & *Keep Moving* is in the integration of the various components into a whole-school approach.

The charts that follow offer a guide to integrating the various fourth- and fifth-grade education components. It is important to remember that this is only a guide. The best way to integrate the program may differ from school to school, depending on each school's particular situation.

Grade 4—Implementation Grid

Classroom Lessons	Promotions	Eat Well Cards and Keep Moving Cards	Physical Education Lessons	Cafeteria	Parent Involvement
1. Healthy Living and the Pyramid			Five Foods Countdown		
2. Energy Foods in the Pyramid	Pyramid Power Game	"The Power of Pasta"	Musical Fare		Reprint Eat Well card in parent newsletter
3. The Safe Workout: An Introduction		"Be Wise . . . Warm-Up for 5 Before You Exercise"			Reprint Keep Moving card in parent newsletter
4. Balancing Act					
5. Fast-Food Frenzy					
6. Snack Attack			Bowling for Snacks		Reprint Keep Moving card in parent newsletter
7. The Safe Workout: Snacking's Just Fine, If You Choose the Right Kind			Three Kinds of Fitness Fun		
8. Prime-Time Smartness	Freeze My TV	"A Piece of the Pie"			Reprint Keep Moving card in parent newsletter
9. Chain-Five	Get 3-at-School & 5-A-Day	"...5-A-Day Should Be Your Goal" "A Juicy Quiz" "Have You Ever Heard of . . . " "Oranges for Each Day's Journey"	Fruits and Vegetables	Dole Foods' "Jammin' 5 A Day Songs" played in cafeteria	Reprint Eat Well cards in parent newsletter
10. Alphabet Fruit (and Vegetables)					
11. Brilliant Breakfast					
12. Fitness Walking	Class-Walking Clubs				

Grade 5—Implementation Grid

Classroom Lessons	Promotions	Eat Well Cards and Keep Moving Cards	Physical Education Lessons	Cafeteria	Parent Involvement
13. Healthy Living and the Pyramid	Pyramid Power Game		Five Foods Countdown		
14. Keeping the Balance					
15. The Safe Workout: A Review		"Be Wise . . . Warm-Up for 5 Before You Exercise"			Reprint Keep Moving card in parent newsletter
16. Hunting for Hidden Fat		"The Power of Pasta"			
17. Snack Decisions			Musical Fare		
18. Snacking and Inactivity		"A Piece of the Pie"	Bowling for Snacks		Reprint Keep Moving card in parent newsletter
19. Freeze My TV	Freeze My TV				Reprint excerpt from *Freeze My TV Journal* in parent newsletter
20. Menu Monitoring					
21. The Game of Veggiemania	Get 3-at-School & 5-A-Day	"...5-A-Day Should Be Your Goal" "A Juicy Quiz" "Have You Ever Heard of . . . " "Oranges for Each Day's Journey"	Fruits and Vegetables	Dole Foods' "Jammin' 5 A Day Songs" played in cafeteria	Reprint Eat Well cards in parent newsletter
22. Breakfast Bonanza					
23. Foods From Around the World					
24. Fitness Walking	Class-Walking Clubs		Three Kinds of Fitness Fun		

Nutrition and Physical Activity Lessons and Promotions

Classroom Lessons for Fourth Graders

The classroom lessons on nutrition and physical activity comprise the cornerstone of Eat Well & *Keep Moving*. Using a multidisciplinary teaching approach, the lessons contained in part I equip students with the knowledge and skills they need to choose a nutritious diet and be physically active both now and throughout their lives. Though effective on their own, these classroom lessons also serve as a springboard for all the other activities of Eat Well & *Keep Moving*—the promotions (part III), physical education lessons (part IV), FitCheck physical education micro-units (part VI), additional physical education micro-units (part VII), and the cafeteria and parent involvement components described in the CD-ROM.

Part I includes the fourth-grade lessons, with which students learn to

- eat at least five servings of fruits and vegetables a day,
- eat less fat (especially saturated and *trans* fats),
- eat a nutritious breakfast every morning,
- be more physically active, and
- be less physically inactive (specifically, reducing time spent viewing television).

Using subject matter areas ranging from language arts to mathematics, these lessons address, among other topics, overall health, the Food Guide Pyramid, smart snacking, and how to perform physical workouts safely.

Healthy Living and the Pyramid

Background

Healthy Living

Healthy living involves making lifestyle choices that maximize your physical and mental well-being. Healthy living encompasses more than just eating a balanced diet. It also involves getting the exercise and rest your body needs to stay healthy, as well as engaging in activities that you enjoy and that enhance your mental well-being.

It is important to recognize that your physical health and your mental health are interrelated. For example: exercising and eating a balanced diet that is low in saturated and trans fat can help maintain a healthy weight, boost mental health by increasing energy levels, and improve your ability to cope with stress. Spending time with friends can help provide support for the many challenges in life as well as provide companions for physical activity. The key to healthy living is a balance of all aspects of life—the physical, intellectual, social, and emotional.

Eating a balanced diet is an important component of a healthy lifestyle. Eating the right foods provides you with the energy and nutrients your body needs to stay healthy and helps fight and prevent some infections and diseases. What you eat not only affects how your body performs and feels today, it also affects your health for 10, 20, 30 years and beyond.

The Food Guide Pyramid

Over the years, experts have worked to form guidelines to help Americans eat better, to keep us healthier, and to enhance quality of life. The Food Guide Pyramid—a concept developed by the United States Department of Agriculture (USDA)—represents years of research on what a healthy diet should consist of for Americans over two years of age.

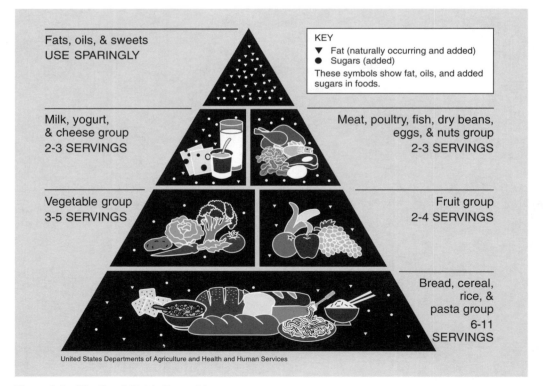

Figure 1.1 The Food Guide Pyramid.

This research focused on what foods Americans eat now, what nutrients are in the foods we eat, and how these patterns need to change to better prevent disease and promote good health. The Food Guide Pyramid emphasizes moderation, variety, and balance. The pyramid helps you choose what and how much to eat from each food group to get the nutrients you need without getting too many calories or too much saturated and *trans* fat, sugar, or sodium. It also helps you to get a good amount of fiber, which is important to your health.

There are six categories in the pyramid, and the size of each category corresponds to the amount of food from that group that we need to eat each day. The groups at the bottom of the pyramid take up more space, which means that we need more of these foods. The food group at the tip of the pyramid is for food items that consist primarily of fat and sugar, demonstrating that it is healthy to eat these only in small amounts. For instance, a diet low in saturated and *trans* fat may help reduce the risk of developing heart disease and some types of cancer.

Table 1.1 Examples of Food Items That Belong in Each Food Group

Food Group	Food Items
Grains (especially whole grains)	bread (corn bread, muffins, rolls, whole wheat bread, tortillas, biscuits, pitas, pancakes, pretzels), cereal, oatmeal, rice, and pasta (macaroni, spaghetti)
Vegetables	collard greens, mustard greens, spinach, kale, corn, turnips, lima beans, string beans, cabbage, white potatoes, sweet potatoes, broccoli, carrots, okra, squash
Fruit	peaches, nectarines, cantaloupe, watermelon, grapefruit, raisins, apples, oranges, bananas, strawberries, pears, tangerines, grapes, pineapple
Meat, Poultry, Fish, Dry Beans, Eggs, & Nuts	peanut butter, kidney beans, navy beans, lentils, black-eyed peas, peanuts, lean meat, chicken, turkey, fish, eggs, tofu
Dairy	nonfat milk, 1% milk, 2% milk, cottage cheese, cheddar cheese, low-fat cheese, frozen yogurt

Estimated Teaching Time and Related Subject Area

Estimated teaching time: 1 hour, 10 minutes

Related subject area: social studies

Objectives

1. Students will understand the concept of healthy living.
2. Students will learn about the Food Guide Pyramid and why its shape is important for a healthy diet.

Materials

1. Worksheet #1, "Origami Pyramid"
2. Worksheet #2, "Help! You're the Doctor"
3. Worksheet #3, "The Doctor Says"
4. Solutions to worksheet #2
5. Solutions to worksheet #3

Procedure

1. Discuss experiences in the everyday life of an urban person—buses, trains, restaurants, busy streets, supermarkets, high-rise buildings, noise pollution. Ask students how the lifestyle of an office worker in the city differs from a farmer's lifestyle in a rural area. Have students discuss the similarities and differences of these lifestyles. Record their answers on the board. If time allows, you may also include the suburban lifestyle in the compare-and-contrast discussion.

   The following chart provides examples of the possible differences between urban and rural lifestyles:

Table 1.2   Urban and Rural Lifestyles

Urban Office Worker	Rural Farmer
takes bus to work	walks to fields
sits at desk all day	works in barn and fields all day
secure job and pay check	pay dependent on nature
eats fast food at lunch	brings lunch from home
buys fruits and vegetables at corner market	buys fruits and vegetables from produce stand
lives close to friends and family	must travel long distance to see friends and family
noisy surroundings	quiet surroundings
many recreational activities easily accessible (movies, concerts, sports)	many recreational activities not easily accessible

2. Discuss with students how people's lifestyles vary a great deal, and that lifestyle can affect a person's health. With the help of the students, list on the board all the things we do to stay healthy—exercise, rest, sleep, eat right, bathe, clean our living and work environments, visit the doctor for check-ups, try to be safe, etc.
3. Distribute worksheet #1, "Origami Pyramid." Provide each student with the Origami Pyramid worksheet and have students assemble the pyramid. Discuss the Food Guide Pyramid concept and food groups with students.
4. Reiterate that it is important to eat more foods from the base and middle of the pyramid and fewer foods from the top of the pyramid.
5. Explain to students that "healthy living" involves ensuring their lifestyle is balanced and varied. Tell them that it is important to eat a balanced and varied diet and to engage in a variety of activities in all aspects of their lives—social,

intellectual, physical, and emotional. For example, this would include activities such as spending time with friends, reading, talking with family members, walking, dancing, running, playing sports, and even having some quiet time. Have students illustrate activities they can choose that will ensure that their lifestyles are varied and balanced.

6. Distribute worksheet #2, "Help! You're the Doctor." Have students read about the people with health concerns and answer the questions in the spaces provided on the worksheet. Discuss answers with the class.

7. Distribute worksheet #3, "The Doctor Says." Based on recommendations in the Food Guide Pyramid, have students suggest some foods that the people discussed in worksheet #2 should consider including in their diet.

Origami Pyramid

Directions

1. Using scissors, cut out the entire origami figure by cutting along the outside lines. Be sure to cut around the two round tabs at the top.

2. Fold the paper so that it forms the shape of a pyramid, and tape the round tabs on the inside of the pyramid to hold it together.

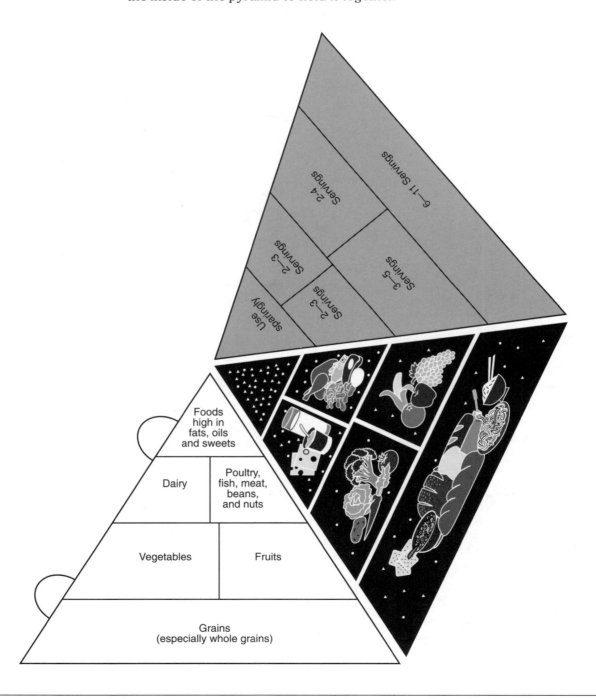

Help! You're the Doctor

Directions

Read the following paragraphs and solve the problems that follow:

> Mr. Jones lives in the city with his wife, son, and two daughters. He works at a local bank that is two miles away from his house, and catches the bus to the office at 8:00 each morning. He usually eats lunch at one of the five fast-food places or restaurants that are on the same street as the bank. After work, he catches the bus home and then watches television after dinner in the evenings. His family is concerned because he has recently put on a lot of weight and does not have much energy to enjoy weekend outdoor activities.

List some suggestions that will help Mr. Jones lose weight and feel more energetic.

_____

_____

_____

_____

_____

_____

_____

> Susan is a fourth-grade student who enjoyed playing basketball last season for the school team. This year she has decided not to play because she spends all her free time on the school's computer. She snacks on candy while she sits. She's becoming less active, and her bedroom is a real mess. Her friends are getting annoyed with her because they never see her anymore.

Explain why it is important for Susan to think about her current lifestyle. Give four suggestions that will help Susan change her current lifestyle.

_____

_____

_____

_____

Worksheet 2

Kyle is 14 years old. He eats a lot of potato chips during the week, but never has the same amount of energy as his friends. On Saturday mornings he enjoys cycling with his friends on a bike trail. He never eats breakfast, however, and is often exhausted after just 10 minutes of cycling. In contrast, his friends drink water and eat nutritious snacks like raisins, crackers, and yogurt. By the end of the morning, they seem less tired than Kyle.

Give some reasons you think will explain why Kyle's energy level is low. What are the two ways Kyle can increase his energy level?

_____

_____

_____

_____

_____

The Doctor Says

Just as you need a variety of activities in your life, you also need a variety of foods. The Food Guide Pyramid divides the foods we eat into six categories and helps us to know how much of each category we need to eat to stay healthy.

Directions

Help Mr. Jones, Susan, and Kyle learn about foods that will benefit their health by completing the exercises below.

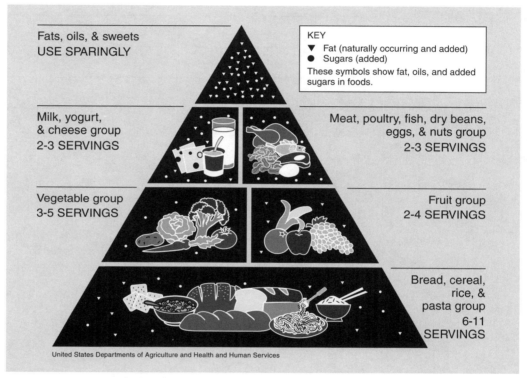

Figure 1.3 The Food Guide Pyramid.

1. Using the Food Guide Pyramid, plan a lunch menu for Mr. Jones for the next workweek. You can decide if he takes his lunch from home or buys it at a store or restaurant.

Monday

_____

Tuesday

_____

Wednesday

_____

Thursday

_____

Friday

_____

Worksheet

3

2. Choose five snacks Susan could eat that would be better for her than candy:

Doughnut	Doritos	Apple
100% fruit juice	Piece of toast	Grapes
Chocolate chip cookies	Gatorade	Fig Newtons
Soda	Low-salt pretzels	Low-fat yogurt
Peach	Banana	Low-fat cheese
Twinkies	Kool-Aid	Cereal

3. List some healthy food choices Kyle should consider for his weekend breakfast.

_____

_____

_____

_____

Solutions

Worksheet 2   Help! You're the Doctor

1. There are many things Mr. Jones could do to help control his weight and feel more energetic. For example:

   Mr. Jones could walk the two miles to and/or from work instead taking the bus.

   Mr. Jones could get off the bus a few stops early and walk the rest of the way.

   He could eat less frequently at the fast-food restaurants and bring a nutritious lunch from home.

   He could choose alternatives that have vegetables (for example, salads, pizza with vegetable topping) at the fast-food restaurants.

   He could go for a walk at lunch.

   He could walk to a restaurant that is farther away than the nearby, fast-food places.

   Instead of watching television over the entire evening, Mr. Jones could also do something more physically active, such as play a sport or join a gym, play with his children, do household chores, and even garden.

2. Susan should be concerned about her new lifestyle for a number of reasons:

   By spending all of her free time on the computer, Susan is becoming very inactive.

   By giving up the basketball team, she is giving up an opportunity to be active, as well as an opportunity to be with friends and learn about the importance of teamwork.

   Susan is letting her obsession with the computer affect other important parts of her life like spending time with friends, being physically active, and even cleaning her room.

   By eating so much candy, Susan is not getting the balanced and varied diet that is so important for energy, growth, and health. On top of this, all those sweets will also greatly increase her chances of cavities. Candy is a nutrient-sparse food containing a lot of calories but not many nutrients.

3. Kyle's energy levels are low because he skips breakfast and eats unhealthy snacks. To increase his energy levels, Kyle should be sure to eat breakfast—ideally a meal that is high in carbohydrates and whole grains, has some protein, and is low in saturated and *trans* fat and sugars. Also, eating nutritious snacks and drinking a lot of water like his friends will give him more energy as the morning of cycling wears on.

Solutions

Worksheet 3 The Doctor Says

1. Using the Food Guide Pyramid, plan a lunch menu for Mr. Jones for the next workweek. You can decide if he takes his lunch from home or buys it at a store or restaurant.

   Sample lunch menus:

   Monday: ham sandwich with lettuce and tomatoes on whole wheat bread, raw carrots, banana, and raisins (with lunch or for snack)

   Tuesday: cold spaghetti with vegetables, mixed tossed salad with a *small amount* (1 tablespoon) of salad dressing, whole wheat roll, apple, and grapes (with lunch or for snack)

   Wednesday: turkey sandwich on whole wheat bread, vegetable soup (in thermos), 1/2 cantaloupe, and low-fat yogurt (with lunch or for snack)

   Thursday: leftover tuna casserole, romaine lettuce or spinach salad with a *small amount* (1 tablespoon) of dressing, strawberries, and a banana (with lunch or for snack)

   Friday: tuna sandwich with a *small amount* of mayonnaise, lettuce and tomatoes, lentil/pea soup (in thermos), pear, and a peach (with lunch or for snack)

2. **Good snack choices:** grapes, banana, apple, peach, 100% fruit juice, low-fat yogurt, piece of toast, low-salt pretzels, Fig Newtons, cereal, and low-fat cheese

   Less healthful snack choices: doughnut, Doritos, chocolate chip cookies, soda, Gatorade, Kool-Aid, and Twinkies

3. Sample healthy breakfast food choices for Kyle:

   Bowl of mixed fruit

   100% orange juice

   Hot oatmeal with fruit

   Melon/cantaloupe with yogurt

   Low-fat granola

   Whole grain cereal with 1% or skim milk

   English muffin with jam

   Banana

   Peaches with 1% or skim milk

   100% tomato juice

   Pancakes with strawberries

   100% grapefruit juice

   Nuts

Energy Foods in the Pyramid

Background

Nutrients

The foods we eat contain many kinds of nutrients. Nutrients are the chemical substances in food that your body uses to keep healthy. Macronutrients (carbohydrates, fats, and proteins) are the major food components. Micronutrients (vitamins and minerals) are the nutrients that you need in very small amounts and are present in many foods. Both groups of nutrients are important for a healthy body.

All foods are made up of one, two, or all three of the macronutrients. The functions of each are described below:

Protein provides the body with the building blocks for making and repairing tissue and helps your body grow (like muscle, bone, hair, and skin). Enzymes that control all the body processes from growth to digestion are also made of protein.

Fat helps keep the body warm, helps protect the internal organs (like the heart and liver), helps the body transport certain vitamins, and is a rich source of energy.

Carbohydrates provide the body with the quickest source of energy. They are the only nutrient that can be readily used for energy in every single cell in the body. Carbohydrates should be the largest part of each day's total food intake in a healthy diet.

Carbohydrates are found in many foods and in all groups of the Food Guide Pyramid. The grain, fruit, and vegetable groups contain the greatest amount of carbohydrates, fiber, vitamins, and minerals. Other good sources include milk, yogurt, and dried beans (legumes). Sweet foods such as soda, cookies, and candy that contain sugar also provide carbohydrate; but, unfortunately, these foods usually contain very little of the micronutrients (vitamins and minerals) and can be high in saturated and *trans* fats. These foods should be eaten only in small amounts on a regular basis.

Estimated Teaching Time and Related Subject Area

Estimated teaching time: 50 minutes

Related subject area: health

Objectives

1. Students will be introduced to the role of carbohydrates in the diet.
2. Students will gain a greater understanding of the Food Guide Pyramid's food groups and serving recommendations.

Materials

1. Food Guide Pyramid poster (sketched by teacher on poster board or butcher paper)

2. Strong tape
3. Food picture cards (often available through your state's Dairy Council) *or* pictures of food cut out from magazines (be sure to include vegetables, fruits, whole grain breads and cereals, and dairy products, which are high in carbohydrates)
4. Worksheet #1, "Which Group?"
5. Worksheet #2, "Carbohydrates—Energy Foods!!"
6. Worksheet #3, "Fueling Up the Body"
7. Teacher Resource Page #1, "Carbohydrate Foods"
8. Teacher Resource Page #2, "Low-Carbohydrate Foods"
9. Solutions to worksheet #1
10. Solutions to worksheet #2
11. Solutions to worksheet #3

Procedure

1. Distribute worksheet #1, "Which Group?" Review the Food Guide Pyramid food groups with students. Have students identify the food groups for each of the foods listed on the worksheet by writing each of them in the spaces provided.

2. Explain to students that this lesson introduces carbohydrates, which are one of three kinds of nutrients in foods that provide us with energy. Carbohydrates (especially in the form of whole grains) should be the main source of energy we get each day, and some foods have more carbohydrates than others. Fat and protein are the other two sources of energy, but carbohydrates should provide the base of energy. Whole grain breads and cereals, beans, fruits, vegetables, and low-fat dairy products are good sources of carbohydrates.

   Teacher Resource Page #1 provides examples of carbohydrate foods. Use this list to ensure that students have selected foods high in carbohydrates for the activity below. Teacher Resource Page #2 lists foods that are *not* rich in carbohydrates.

3. Place the Food Guide Pyramid poster on the wall and spread all the food picture cards on the floor or a large table. Have students individually select foods that are good sources of carbohydrates and place them next to the appropriate food group on the wall. Another option is to have sections of the room represent different food groups. Students can then move to the section of the room that corresponds to the food group to which their high-carbohydrate choice belongs. Next, have all students write the foods selected in the food group boxes on worksheet #2. All food groups should be represented, since there are high-carbohydrate choices available in each group.

4. Have students form groups and complete worksheet #3, "Fueling Up the Body," which involves planning a menu for a physically active individual of their choice. They can choose an Olympic athlete, a professional dancer, a basketball star, a friend who plays a lot of sports, or even themselves.

1 Which Group?

Directions

Write each of the foods listed in the table below in the boxes under the appropriate food group in the next table. You will need to put more than one item in each box, so please write small enough to include many food items.

Table 2.1

Bananas	Sweet potatoes	Macaroni	Sunflower seeds
Apples	Broccoli	Margarine	Whole grain rolls
Brown rice	Squash	Butter	Cheese
Whole grain bread	Low-fat cheese	Lettuce	Pancakes
Spaghetti	Candy	Cabbage	Walnuts
Low-fat milk	Peaches	Greens	Nonfat milk
Low-fat yogurt	Low-fat pudding	Kale	Grapes
Coca-Cola	Bacon	Tortillas	Chicken
Oatmeal	Cheerios	Baked beans	Kool-Aid
Strawberries	Corn	Spinach	Carrots
Peanut butter	Hominy grits	Blueberries	Watermelon
Black-eyed peas	Oranges	Turkey	Eggs
Ice milk	Tuna	Cottage cheese	Plums
Salad dressing	Lean roast beef	Gravy	Low-fat chocolate milk
Potato chips	Buttermilk	Kiwi fruit	Low-fat cream cheese

Table 2.2   Food Groups

Grains	Vegetables	Fruits	Beans, Meat, & Fish	Dairy	Fats, Oils, & Sweets
		Example: Bananas			

Worksheet 2

Carbohydrates— Energy Foods!!

Directions

Write each of the high-carbohydrate foods that the class selects in the correct food group box below.

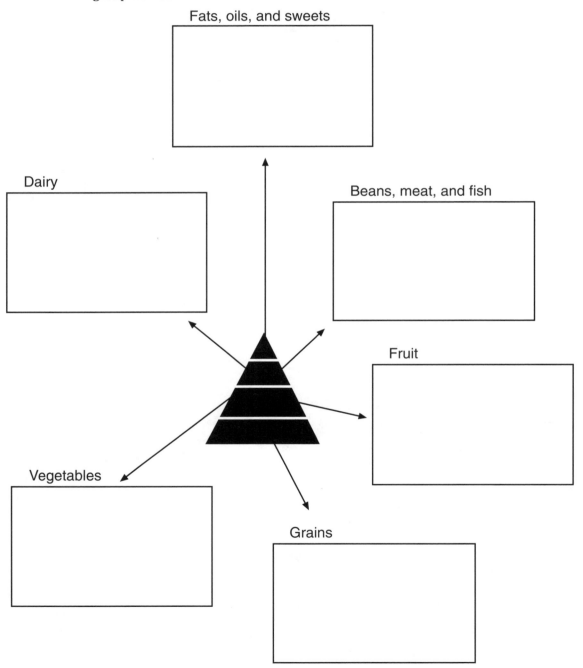

Fats, oils, and sweets

Dairy

Beans, meat, and fish

Fruit

Vegetables

Grains

Fueling Up the Body

My name_____

Other group members_____

Directions

As a group, pick an athlete or very active person who needs a lot of energy. You don't have to pick a superathlete; it can even be someone's friend or family member. Next, plan a day's menu for the person. Remember to choose a lot of energy foods and make sure it follows the Food Guide Pyramid.

Person's name_____

Breakfast

_____

Lunch

_____

Snack

_____

Dinner

_____

Snack

_____

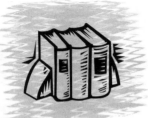

Teacher Resource Page #1

Carbohydrate Foods

Examples of foods that are good sources of carbohydrates:

Baked potato	Linguini/macaroni	Pinto beans
Banana	Skim or 1% milk	Plantains
Black beans	Low-fat yogurt	Plums
Black-eyed peas	Mango	Polenta
Brown rice	Mashed potatoes	Pretzels
Corn	Navy beans	Raisin bread
Cornflakes	Nectarines	Rice
Couscous	Oatmeal	Spaghetti
Cream of wheat	Oatmeal raisin cookies	Squash
French bread	Orange juice	Sweet potatoes
Garbanzo beans	Oranges	Waffles
Grapes	Pancakes	Whole grain cereal
Green beans	Peaches	Whole wheat bread
Lima beans	Pears	

Teacher Resource Page #2

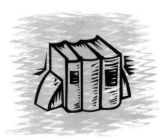

Low-Carbohydrate Foods

Examples of foods that are *not* high in carbohydrates:

Meat	Fish
Hamburger (without bun)	Eggs
Hot dog (without bun)	Cucumbers
Cheese	Mushrooms
Lettuce	Greens
Celery	Nuts
Chicken	

Solutions

Worksheet 1   Which Group?

Directions

Write each of the foods in the boxes under the appropriate food group.

Table 2.4   Food Groups

Grains	Vegetables	Fruits	Beans, Meat, & Fish	Dairy	Fats, Oils, & Sweets
Brown rice	Broccoli	Bananas	Peanut butter	Low-fat milk	Coca-Cola
Whole grain bread	Squash	Apples	Black-eyed peas	Low-fat yogurt	Salad dressing
Spaghetti	Corn	Strawberries	Tuna	Ice milk	Potato chips
Oatmeal	Lettuce	Peaches	Lean roast beef	Buttermilk	Candy
Cheerios	Cabbage	Oranges	Baked beans	Cottage cheese	Low-fat pudding
Hominy grits	Greens	Blueberries	Turkey	Cheese	Bacon
Macaroni	Kale	Kiwi fruit	Walnuts	Low-fat chocolate milk	Margarine
Tortillas	Spinach	Grapes	Chicken	Low-fat cream cheese	Butter
Whole grain rolls	Carrots	Watermelon	Eggs	Nonfat milk	Gravy
Pancakes	Sweet potatoes	Plums	Sunflower seeds	Low-fat cheese	Kool-Aid

Solutions

Worksheet 2   Carbohydrates–Energy Foods!!

Directions

Write each of the foods that the class selects in the correct food group box below.

Fats, oils, and sweets

Sodas, cookies, and most candy have a lot of carbohydrates but contain very little vitamins and minerals. They therefore, should not be consumed very often.

Dairy

Low-fat milk
Low-fat yogurt

Beans, meat, and fish

Black beans
Black-eyed peas
Garbanzo beans
Navy beans
Pinto beans

Fruit

Banana	Pears
Blackberries	Plantains
Blueberries	Plums
Grapes	Strawberries
Mango	
Nectarines	
Orange juice	

Vegetables

Baked potato	Squash
Lima beans	Corn
Green beans	
Sweet potatoes	
Mashed potatoes	

Grains

Baked potato	Raisin bread
Cereal	French bread
Cornflakes	Cream of wheat
Couscous	Whole wheat
Rice	bread
Polenta	Spaghetti
Oatmeal	Waffles
Pancakes	

Solutions

Worksheet 3   Fueling Up the Body

My name _____

Other group members _____

Directions

As a group, pick an athlete or very active person who needs a lot of energy. You don't have to pick a superathlete; it can even be someone's friend or family member. Next, plan a day's menu for the person. Remember to choose a lot of energy foods and make sure it follows the Food Guide Pyramid.

Person's name ___Marion Jones_____

Breakfast	Cheerios with nonfat milk (2 servings grain, 1 serving dairy), 100% orange juice (1 serving fruit), 1 banana (1 serving fruit)
Lunch	Turkey sandwich on whole wheat bread (1 serving meat, 2 servings grain), strawberry low-fat yogurt (1 serving dairy), 1 apple (1 serving fruit)
Snack	Low-fat fig bars (1 serving grain), carrot sticks (1 serving vegetable)
Dinner	Large plate of spaghetti with red sauce (2 servings grain, 1 serving vegetable), whole wheat French bread (1 serving grain), large helping of steamed broccoli (2 servings vegetable), green salad with white beans (1 serving vegetable, 1 serving beans)
Snack	Banana (1 serving fruit), cup of nonfat milk (1 serving dairy)

The Safe Workout: An Introduction

Background

The human body can do amazing things. However, in order for the body to perform well it must be taken care of. To keep their bodies healthy, people must choose good foods, exercise regularly, stay away from harmful substances (such as tobacco and drugs), and get plenty of sleep. The body uses good food for energy, growth, and repairing itself. Exercising regularly helps keep the body healthy. Some exercises make the heart, lungs, and blood vessels stronger. Some exercises help with flexibility and the body's ability to bend. Some exercises help maintain a healthy weight. The body needs all kinds of exercise. This lesson will teach students the safe way to exercise and at the same time review the Food Guide Pyramid. The pyramid was developed to help individuals choose a balanced and varied diet.

This lesson introduces the five parts of a safe workout. These five parts are important to help prevent injuries while exercising. The five parts of a safe workout are (1) the warm-up, (2) the stretch, (3) the fitness activity, (4) the cool-down, and (5) the cool-down stretch. Each part will be introduced by stating why it is important and how to do it correctly. Because of time constraints, the parts of the lesson workout are shorter than what they normally should be in an actual workout. For example, the lesson warm-up is only one to two minutes long, when ideally the warm-up should be at least five minutes. What's important is that the students learn that a warm-up is the first part of a safe workout and that it should be done at home before they exercise on their bikes or play basketball.

Exercising and doing the five parts of a safe workout is only half of the story! In addition to being physically active, eating right is the other half of the winning combination that keeps our bodies healthy. The students will be learning about the Food Guide Pyramid while moving!

This is a classroom-based activity that can be used as a practice lesson for the other physical activity lessons that will be done in the gymnasium, community room, or cafeteria.

Overview

This lesson introduces students to the various parts of a safe workout. Students, as a class, review the different workout components and then form groups, with each group presenting a different part of the workout to the entire class. At the heart of this lesson is a fitness-activity game in which students gather foods that constitute a balanced meal based on the Food Guide Pyramid.

Estimated Teaching Time and Related Subject Area

Estimated teaching time: 1 hour, 20 minutes

Related subject area: physical education

Objectives

1. Students will be able to identify and sequence the components of a safe and healthy workout.
2. Students will discuss and demonstrate each component of a safe workout.

3. Students will demonstrate awareness of the food groups that make up the Food Guide Pyramid.

Materials

1. Pictures of various foods
2. Food Guide Pyramid outline
3. An information card defining and describing each of the components of a safe workout, why each is important, and an example of an exercise that represents the component (provided)
4. Five information cards, one for each of the food groups in the Food Guide Pyramid, with examples of foods found in the particular group on each card: grain; fruit; vegetable; dairy; and meat, fish, poultry, and dry bean group (provided)
5. Stretching and Strength Fitness diagrams (see appendix, pp. 453-459)
6. Sentence strips for each part of a safe workout and the key terms that relate to various aspects of fitness (provided)

Procedure

1. Each component of the safe workout is written on an individual sentence strip.

   The warm-up (1-2 minutes)

   The stretch (1-2 minutes)

   The fitness activity (15-20 minutes)

   The cool-down (1 minute)

   The cool-down stretch (1 minute)

2. Randomly scatter the sentence strips with the components of the safe workout on the left side of the black board.

   Warm-up: the first part of the safe workout, in which slow movements get the body ready for stretching and the fitness activity.

   Stretch: the part of the safe workout in which you do exercises that improve flexibility fitness and get the body ready for the fitness activity.

   Fitness activity: the part of a safe workout in which strength and endurance fitness exercises are performed.

   Cool-down: the part of the safe workout in which your body slows down and recovers from the fitness activity.

   Cool-down stretch: the last part of the safe workout in which you do exercises that improve flexibility fitness.

3. On the right side of the blackboard, place the sentence strips that contain key fitness terms relating to the components of the workout.

   Pacing: maintaining a comfortable speed so that you can perform your exercise over an extended period of time.

   Flexibility fitness: the part of fitness that stretches the muscles and parts around the muscles to get your body ready for action.

Strength fitness: the part of fitness that makes your muscles, except the heart muscle, stronger and healthier.

Endurance fitness: the part of fitness that improves the heart muscle, lungs, and blood vessels and that helps maintain weight.

4. As a class, read aloud all the terms on the board.

5. Ask the students: "Who knows the first step of a safe workout?" Have a student come to the board to answer the question. After the student gives the correct answer, let the student select the "warm-up" sentence strip and place it on an open part of the blackboard.

6. Continue by asking, "What is the second step of a safe workout?" Another student answers, picks the "stretch" strip, and puts it on the board in the correct order— just after the "warm-up" strip. Repeat this process for the remaining components of the workout.

7. After the workout is in order, discuss the terms: flexibility fitness, strength fitness, endurance fitness, and pacing. Ask the students where they think each term should be placed in the workout (for example: "flexibility fitness" belongs with the "stretch" component of the workout). Have the students provide the answer and then place the term with the appropriate component of the workout.

8. Provide a short introduction to the lesson: "We learned that it is important for our bodies to get the right amounts and kinds of food daily. We also learned that we should eat a variety of different foods and that we should eat foods from all of the different groups represented in the pyramid. The Food Guide Pyramid is a chart that we use as a guide to help us learn to eat foods that will help our bodies stay healthy, grow, and perform physical activities like playing and dancing. The Food Guide Pyramid lets us know how making the right choices about the food we eat affects the health of our bodies. Regular, moderate to vigorous physical activity is also important to our body's health. Just as the Food Guide Pyramid steers us in the right direction so that we eat foods that make us healthy, the safe workout steers us in the right direction so that we exercise and participate in physical activities in ways that are good for our bodies."

9. Have the class form five groups and give each group the name of one of the five food groups from the Food Guide Pyramid. Give each group the "Food Group Information Card" with the name of their food group and examples of the foods found in that group. Equal numbers of students will be represented in the grain group; fruit group; vegetable group; dairy group; and the meat, fish, and dry bean group. Tell students that you (the teacher) will represent the tip of the Pyramid: fats, oils, and sweets. Ask students to provide examples of the foods you represent. Then, remind them that these foods are to be used sparingly.

Grain group includes whole grain breads (corn bread, muffins, rolls, whole wheat bread, biscuits, pancakes, pretzels), whole grain cereal, rice, oatmeal, and pasta (macaroni, spaghetti).

Vegetable group includes collard greens, mustard greens, spinach, kale, corn, turnips, lima beans, string beans, cabbage, white potatoes, sweet potatoes, broccoli, carrots, okra, squash.

Fruit group includes peaches, nectarines, cantaloupes, watermelons, grapefruits, raisins, apples, oranges, bananas, strawberries, pears.

Dry beans, eggs, nuts, fish, and meat and poultry group includes peanut butter, kidney beans, navy beans, black-eyed peas, peanuts, lean meat, chicken, turkey, beef, fish, eggs.

Dairy group includes milk (skim milk, 1% milk, 2% milk, whole milk), cottage cheese, cheddar cheese, American cheese, yogurt, frozen yogurt.

Tell students, "When eating, we must be sure to put the different combinations of foods together in a particular way so that we can have a balanced and nutritious meal. When doing physical activity, we must do different kinds of things so that we can have a safe and beneficial workout. The safe workout can be broken into five parts. We will discuss and go through each of these parts so that you understand what they are and how and when they should be done."

10. Randomly give each group of students a safe workout card defining and describing a component of the workout. Each card names the component, explains why it is important, and gives an example of an exercise that could be done to represent that component. The first three components—warm-up, stretch, and fitness (which includes two cards, strength and endurance)—can be distributed as they are; the last two components—the cool-down and the cool-down stretch—can be handed to one group.

11. Allow students from three to five minutes to review their component and the other information on the card among the members of their group. Explain that a speaker from each of the groups will introduce the entire class to the component and lead the class in doing the exercises for the first three components (warm-up, stretch, and fitness activity).

12. Following the order of the safe workout, have a student from the warm-up group and a student from the stretching group introduce their individual component and lead the class in the appropriate exercises. Be sure the speaker from the warm-up group presents before the speaker from the stretching group.

   a. Warm-up

      1. Benefits of warming-up
         - Helps prevent injuries.
         - Increases body temperature.
         - Gets the body ready for the rest of the workout.
      2. How to warm up
         - Perform a series of slow movements for 5-10 minutes.
         - Examples include slow jogging in place, slow jumping jacks.

   b. Stretch

      1. Benefits of stretching
         - Improves flexibility fitness.
         - Improves the ability of muscles to work.
         - Improves the body's ability to move.
         - Decreases the number of injuries.
      2. How to stretch (see photos in appendix, pp. 453-456)
         - Hold stretch for 10 or more seconds (count out loud: 1 Mississippi, 2 Mississippi . . . to 10 Mississippi).
         - Don't bounce, hold stretch gently.
         - Stretch slowly.
         - Use proper form to avoid injuries.
         - Examples: neck stretch, butterfly, quad burner (thigh stretch).

13. After the warm-up and stretching exercises are finished, explain to the students that they are now prepared to complete the fitness components.

14. Have the next two groups introduce the two fitness components and lead the entire class in the exercises.

a. Strength fitness (see photos in appendix, pp. 457-459)

1. Benefits of strength fitness
   - Improves the ability of your muscles to move or resist a force or workload.
   - Helps you perform your daily tasks without getting tired.
   - Helps prevent injuries.
   - Improves your skills in games and sports—e.g., jumping rope, playing dodge ball, shooting a basketball.

2. How to improve strength fitness
   - Make your muscles work more than they are used to—e.g., go faster, go longer, lift heavier objects, exercise more often.
   - Train, don't strain.
   - Not too much, too soon, or too often.

b. Endurance fitness

1. Benefits of endurance fitness
   - Helps improve heart, lungs, and blood-vessel health (cardiovascular fitness).
   - Helps maintain a healthy weight.
   - Gives you energy.

2. How to improve endurance fitness
   - Do nonstop, continuous movement activities—e.g., nonstop bike riding, nonstop walking, nonstop rope jumping (students may jog or walk in place to demonstrate endurance activities in class).
   - Find a pace (speed) you can do for a long time—"Pace, don't race!"
   - As a goal, do endurance activities three to four days a week for 20-30 minutes.
   - Find an endurance activity you like so you will want to do it.

(During this time you should walk around the class and make corrections as the students are doing these exercises).

15. After you have reviewed the fitness components, lead the class in the shopping fitness activity. Point out to the students an area in the room where numerous and various pictures of food from the different food groups are scattered. This is the grocery store. (You can put pictures into place before class begins.)

16. Explain that each group will be responsible for gathering pictures from the store that make up a healthy, well-balanced meal (breakfast, lunch, dinner, or snack) based on the Food Guide Pyramid (see "Gym line formation" on page 36). Students will gather the appropriate food pictures off the floor.

17. Each member of the group will be responsible for finding a food/drink from a particular food group, making sure the item helps to create a balanced meal. If necessary, review with students the recommendations of the Food Guide Pyramid and the importance of gathering more foods from the bottom parts of the pyramid (grains, fruits, vegetables) and fewer from the upper sections (dairy; beans and meat; and fats, oils, and sweets).

18. The students should be actively engaged when doing the fitness activity. Each team will have to jog lightly throughout the entire activity as individuals from each

group go one at a time to the food-picture piles, while fellow team members wait their turn (15 minutes maximum).

19. When the fitness activity is completed, have the last two groups present the cool-down and cool-down stretches, respectively.

    a. Cool-down
       1. Benefits of cooling down
          • Lets the body slow down or recover from the fitness activity.
          • Helps prevent injuries and muscle soreness.
       2. How to cool down
          • Walk slowly.
          • Walk in place slowly.
    b. Cool-down stretch (see the appendix, p. 453-456)
       1. Benefits of the cool-down stretch
          • Helps prevent soreness.
          • Improves flexibility fitness.
       2. How to do the cool-down stretch
          • Hold stretch for 10 or more seconds (count out loud: 1 Mississippi, 2 Mississippi . . . to 10 Mississippi).
          • Examples: neck stretch, butterfly, quad burner (thigh stretch).

20. When the cool-down stretch has been completed, have all of the groups reassemble.

21. Allow each group several minutes to go around and share the healthy meal and foods they have selected with the other groups.

22. When all groups have completed this, have the students complete an individual writing assignment about their healthy meal.

Gym line formation
for shopping fitness activities

[**X** = one student,   ☐ = teacher (fats, oils, and sweets)]

The purpose of the game is to determine if each student in a group knows which food items from the Food Guide Pyramid fit into their food group. We are also playing this game so that we can become fit and learn how to pace ourselves so that we can make our bodies stronger and able to do an activity for a certain length of time without becoming tired.

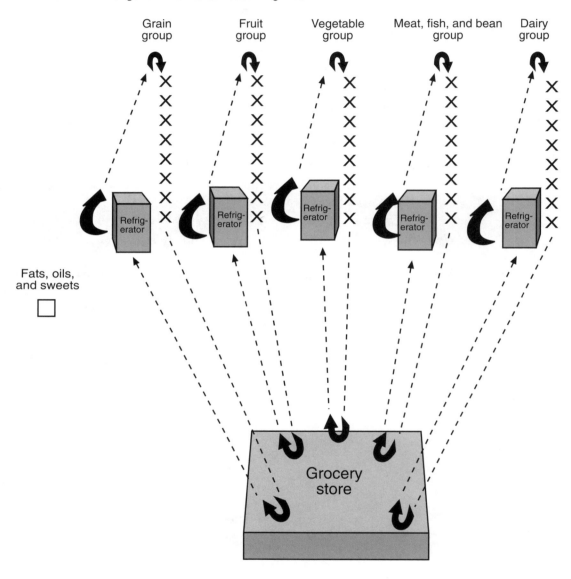

Classroom Line Formation Options

The best option depends on the layout of the classroom.

Option #1

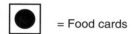= Food cards

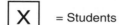= Students

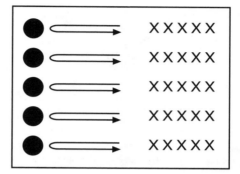

Option #2

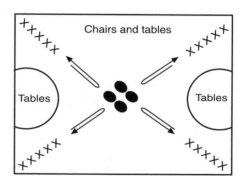

Option #3

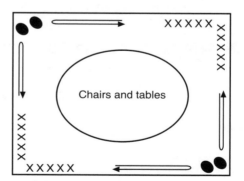

Safe Workout Component Cards

Warm-up

Benefits of warm-up
- Helps prevent injuries.
- Increases body temperature.
- Gets the body ready for the rest of the workout.

How to warm-up
- Perform a series of slow movements for 5–10 minutes
- Examples include slow jogging in place, slow jumping jacks.

Stretch

Benefits of stretching
- Improves flexibility fitness.
- Improves the ability of the muscles to work.
- Improves the body's ability to move.
- Decreases the number of injuries.

How to stretch
- Hold the stretch for 10 or more seconds (count out loud: 1 Mississippi, 2 Mississippi . . . to 10 Mississippi).
- Don't bounce; hold stretch gently.
- Stretch slowly.
- Use proper form to avoid injuries.
- Examples include neck stretch, butterfly, quad burner (thigh stretch).

Strength fitness

Why strength fitness?
- Improves the ability of your muscles to move or resist a force or workload.
- Healthy muscles help you perform your daily tasks without getting tired.
- Helps prevent injuries.
- Improves your skills in games an sports; e.g., jumping rope, playing dodgeball, shooting a basketball.

How to improve strength fitness
- Make your muscles work more than they are used to; e.g., go faster, go longer, lift heavier objects, exercise more often.
- Train, don't strain.
- Don't do too much too soon.
- Examples include push-ups and stomach crunches.

Endurance fitness

Why endurance fitness?
- Helps improve heart, lung, and blood-vessel health (cardiovascular fitness).
- Helps the body maintain a healthy weight.
- Gives you energy.

How to improve endurance fitness
- Do nonstop, continous movement activities; e.g., nonstop bike riding, nonstop walking, nonstop rope jumping.
- Find a pace (speed) you can do for a long time — "pace, don't race!"
- As a goal, do endurance activities 3 to 4 days a week for 20 to 30 minutes.
- Find an endurance activity you like so you will want to do it.

Cool-down

Benefits of cooling down
- Lets the body slow down or recover from the fitness activity.
- Helps prevent injury and muscle soreness.

How to cool-down
- Walk slowly.
- Walk in place slowly.

Cool-down stretch

Benefits of the cool-down stretch
- Helps prevent soreness.
- Improves flexibility fitness.

How to do the cool-down stretch
- Hold the stretch for 10 or more seconds (count our loud: 1 Mississippi, 2 Mississippi . . . to 10 Mississippi).
- Examples include neck stretch, butterfly, quad burner (thigh stretch).

Food Group Information Cards

Grain group

Includes: bread (corn bread, muffins, rolls,
whole wheat bread, biscuits, pancakes, pretzels),
whole grain cereal, rice, and pasta (macaroni, spaghetti)

Vegetable group

Includes: collard greens, mushrooms, tomatoes, peas,
mustard greens, spinach, kale, corn, turnips, lima beans,
string beans, cabbage, white potatoes, sweet potatoes,
broccoli, carrots, okra, squash

Fruit group

Includes: peaches, nectarines, cantaloupe,
watermelon, grapefruit, raisins, apples, oranges,
bananas, strawberries, tangerines

Meat, poultry, fish, dry beans, eggs, and nuts group

includes peanut butter, kidney beans, navy beans,
black-eyed peas, peanuts, lean cuts of
meat, chicken, turkey, beef, fish, eggs

Dairy group

includes nonfat milk, 1% milk, 2% milk,
cottage cheese, low-fat cheese,
yogurt

Components of a Safe Workout

 Sentence Strips

Warm-up: The first part of the safe workout in which slow movements get the body ready for stretching and the fitness activity.

Stretch: The part of the safe workout in which you do exercises that improve flexibility fitness and get the body ready for the fitness activity.

Fitness activity: The part of a safe workout in which you perform strength and endurance fitness exercises.

Cool-down: The part of the safe workout in which your body slows down and recovers from the fitness activity.

Cool-down stretch: The last part of the safe workout in which you do exercises that improve flexibility fitness.

Terms Related to a Safe Workout

 Sentence Strips

Pacing: Maintaining a comfortable speed so that you can perform your exercise over an extended period of time.

Flexibility fitness: The part of fitness that stretches the muscles and parts around the muscles to get your body ready for action.

Strength fitness: The part of fitness that gets your muscles (except the heart muscle) stronger and healthier.

Endurance fitness: The part of fitness that helps improve the heart muscle, lungs, and blood vessels and that helps maintain weight.

Balancing Act

Background

The Food Guide Pyramid provides an excellent example of how to eat a balanced diet every day. People who choose the minimum number of servings from each of the five food groups will get most, if not all, of the nutrients needed to maintain good health.

The GET 3-AT-SCHOOL & 5-A-DAY promotion, which encourages students to eat more fruits and vegetables, can be used as an extension to this lesson. See lesson 26 in part III, Promotions for the Classroom, for details.

A balanced diet is important because different foods contain different combinations of important nutrients. No single food can supply all the nutrients needed to maintain good health. This is why balance and variety go hand in hand. For example, oranges provide vitamin C, but no vitamin B_{12}; cheese provides vitamin B_{12}, but no vitamin C. It is important to remember that foods in one food group cannot replace those in another. Choosing a variety of foods between groups and within groups will help make your diet more interesting, as well as balanced.

Nutrition surveys have found that American children are eating too much saturated fat and not eating enough fruits and vegetables; nor are they getting enough foods that are high in calcium.

Estimated Teaching Time and Related Subject Areas

Estimated teaching time: 80 minutes

Related subject areas: science, math

Objectives

1. Students will learn to discuss the importance of a balanced diet.
2. Students will be able to examine menus and learn to identify and link sources of nutrients with specific foods.

Materials

1. Transparency #1, "Food Guide Pyramid"
2. Transparency #2, "Mary's Menu—Food Choices"
3. Worksheet #1, "Food, Nutrients, and You"
4. Worksheet #2, "Runner's Balanced Diet"
5. Worksheet #3, "Now You Create a Balanced Meal!"
6. Solutions to transparency #2
7. Solutions to worksheet #3

Procedure

1. Ask students to discuss the meaning of the word "balance." Possible student responses:

   - Balance represents equality, fairness.
   - Balance means to remain upright, avoid falling.
   - Balance means to be stable, steady.
   - Balance means that one side equals the other side. There is not too much or too little on either side.

2. Ask the students how the definition of "balance" relates to the term "a balanced diet."

 Key Idea Having a "balanced diet" means *eating a variety of foods from all areas of the Food Guide Pyramid* according to the recommended proportions.

   Possible student responses:

   - The amount of food you eat and the amount of exercise you get need to balance or you'll gain too much weight or lose too much weight.
   - People need to eat different kinds of foods for the body to obtain an assortment of vitamins, minerals, carbohydrates, protein, fats, and water.
   - If you eat one food all the time, you won't get enough of the nutrients provided by other food choices, so you won't be "balanced."

3. Project the Food Guide Pyramid transparency and review with students the number of suggested servings in each group. Next, project the "Mary's Menu—Food Choices" transparency and have students examine Mary's menu to see how many food groups are represented and approximately how many servings of each group are present. Count them up together and fill in the grid on the transparency.

   Ask the students, "Is Mary's diet balanced or unbalanced?" (Answer: It is balanced, but she needs at least two more servings from the grain group to meet the Food Guide Pyramid recommendations. There are approximately four grain foods, three fruits, three vegetables, two meat choices, and three dairy food items. In addition, the cookies fall into the sweets category at the tip of the pyramid.)

4. Review the meaning of the term, "eating balanced meals."

   Key discussion points:

   - It is important to eat a variety of foods from each area of the Food Guide Pyramid because this helps provide your body with a balanced diet. A balanced diet is important because foods in one food group cannot replace those in another group. We need foods from all food groups in order to be healthy.

   - The "suggested number" of servings is a guide that lets us know how important the different food groups are to a healthy body. In looking at the Food Guide Pyramid, we can see that the largest part of the pyramid comprises grains (especially whole grains), fruits, and vegetables. So grains, fruits, and vegetables are very, very important.

   - Eating several servings from the tip of the pyramid (fats, oils, and sweets) and fewer from the bottom three areas (grains, fruits, and vegetables) would not provide your body with a balanced diet. Most people in the United States eat too many foods high in fat and refined sugar from the top part of the pyramid.

5. Distribute the "Food, Nutrients, and You" worksheet and briefly discuss the six types of nutrients, their functions, and their food sources.

6. Have students form pairs or small groups. Distribute worksheet #2 and read "A Runner's Story" aloud.

A Runner's Story

A long-distance runner has been training hard for the past month. She has been running every day and has been eating a balanced diet. She is racing and runs hard toward the finish line. Her training and her balanced diet help her to win the race.

7. After reading the story, have students discuss in their pairs/small groups how specific foods and their related nutrients would help the runner successfully train and complete the race. Have them fill in the blanks on the chart, including what she might have eaten to get each nutrient. (See sample chart on p. 55.)

8. Display the Food Guide Pyramid transparency once again and relate student answers back to the pyramid. From which groups of the pyramid do the foods they picked for the "Runner's Balanced Diet" worksheet come?

Summary

1. Distribute the "Now You Create a Balanced Meal!" worksheet. In their pairs or small groups, have students create a balanced menu. A solutions worksheet is provided as an example.

2. When the pairs/small groups have finished, ask them to share their balanced meals with the class. Post each group's meal on a bulletin board for everyone to view.

3. Encourage the students to ensure that their meals are as balanced as possible each day so they will get all the nutrients they need to grow and be healthy.

The Food Guide Pyramid

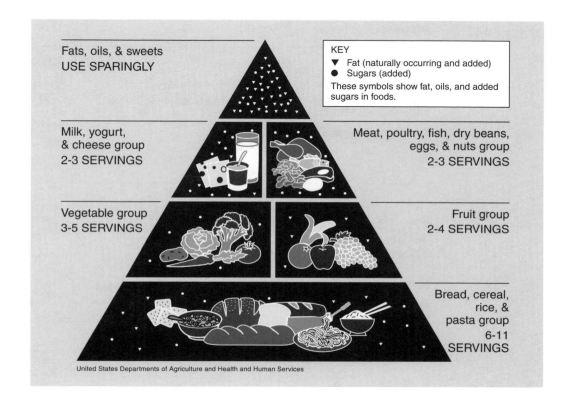

Fats, oils, & sweets
USE SPARINGLY

KEY
▼ Fat (naturally occurring and added)
● Sugars (added)
These symbols show fat, oils, and added sugars in foods.

Milk, yogurt,
& cheese group
2-3 SERVINGS

Meat, poultry, fish, dry beans,
eggs, & nuts group
2-3 SERVINGS

Vegetable group
3-5 SERVINGS

Fruit group
2-4 SERVINGS

Bread, cereal,
rice, &
pasta group
6-11
SERVINGS

United States Departments of Agriculture and Health and Human Services

Mary's Menu— Food Choices

Table 4.1   Mary's Menu—Food Choices

Breakfast	Lunch	Dinner
Banana	Apple	Spinach (1 cup)
Milk	Turkey/lettuce sandwich on 2 slices of whole wheat bread	Baked chicken nuggets (6-8 pieces)
Whole grain cereal	Carrot sticks	Whole wheat roll
100% orange juice	2 cookies	1% milk
	1% milk	

Table 4.2   Food Groups

Food Groups	Recommended Number of Servings	Number of Servings in Mary's Menu
Bread, cereal, rice, and pasta group	6-11	
Vegetable group	3-5	
Fruit group	2-4	
Milk, yogurt, and cheese group	2-3	
Meat, poultry, fish, dry beans, eggs, and nuts group	2-3	
Fats, oils, and sweets	(use sparingly)	

Food, Nutrients, and You

Table 4.3 Food, Nutrients, and You

Nutrient & Functions	Food Sources
Water	
• Helps cool your body when it's working hard • Helps you digest your food • Helps nutrients get to different parts of the body	Water, drinks without caffeine, fruit, soup
Carbohydrates	
• Give you energy • Can be stored as energy for later use • Give sweetness and texture to foods • Provide a good source of vitamins, minerals, and fiber	Whole grains, fruit, starchy and root vegetables (like potatoes, yams, and sweet potatoes)
Minerals	
• Help your blood carry oxygen and nutrients to your muscles and other body parts • Help build strong bones and teeth	Whole grains, lean meat, milk, vegetables, fruit, cheese, legumes (dry beans)
Protein	
• Builds and repairs muscles • Helps your body grow	Meat, poultry, fish, dry beans, nuts, milk and milk products, eggs, tofu
Vitamins	
• Help you to see better at night • Help your body get energy from the food you eat • Help your body heal cuts and bruises • Help you fight off infections	Vegetables, fruit, fish, whole grains, milk and milk products
Fat	
• Gives you energy, especially for long-term use • Makes you feel less hungry • Makes food taste good • Helps keep your skin smooth	Vegetable oil, meats and nuts, milk products (cheese)

Runner's Balanced Diet

A Runner's Story
A long-distance runner has been training hard for the past month. She has been running every day and has been eating a balanced diet. She is racing and runs hard toward the finish. Her training and her balanced diet help her to win the race.

Question: Why does she need to eat a balanced diet, and how did it help her to win? Use the "Food, Nutrients, and You" page to fill out the chart below.

Table 4.4   Runner's Balanced Diet

Nutrients in Her Balanced Diet	How Nutrients Help Her	What She Might Have Eaten
Minerals		
Carbohydrates		
Fat		
Protein		
Vitamins		
Water		

Table 4.5   Example of a Runner's Balanced Diet

Nutrients in Her Balanced Diet	How Nutrients Help Her	What She Might Have Eaten (*examples*)
Minerals	Give runner strong bones Help runner's blood carry oxygen to muscles	Chicken, whole grain bread, 1% milk
Carbohydrates	Give runner quick energy	Pasta, bananas, whole grain bread, fruits
Fat	Gives runner long-term energy	Vegetable oil (in salad dressing and cooking) 1% milk, nuts, granola
Protein	Helps runner build up and repair muscles	1% milk, chicken, beans
Vitamins	Help runner see at night Help runner get energy from food	Carrots, broccoli, spinach, oranges
Water	Helps runner stay cool while she is running hard Helps nutrients get to different parts of the body	Water, fruit juice, vegetable juice, soups, fresh fruit

Now You Create a Balanced Meal!

Directions

Create a balanced meal that you would enjoy. Pick a food from each food group and then write down the nutrients that each food gives you.

Table 4.6 **Now You Create a Balanced Meal!**

Food Group	Your Food Choice	Nutrients Food Gives You
Grains		
Fruits		
Vegetables		
Meat, Poultry, Fish, Dry Beans, Eggs, and Nuts		
Dairy		

Solutions

Transparency 2   Mary's Menu–Food Choices

Table 4.7   Mary's Menu—Food Choices

Breakfast	Lunch	Dinner
Banana	Apple	Spinach (1 cup)
Milk	Turkey/lettuce sandwich on 2 slices of whole wheat bread	Baked chicken nuggets (6-8 pieces)
Whole grain cereal	Carrot sticks	Whole wheat roll
100% orange juice	2 cookies	1% milk
	1% milk	

Table 4.8   Food Groups

Food Groups	Recommended Number of Servings	Number of Servings in Mary's Menu
Bread, cereal, rice, and pasta group	6-11	4
Vegetable group	3-5	3
Fruit group	2-4	3
Milk, yogurt, and cheese group	2-3	3
Meat, poultry, fish, dry beans, eggs, and nuts group	2-3	2
Fats, oils, and sweets	(use sparingly)	2

Solutions

Worksheet 3   Now You Create a Balanced Meal!

Directions

Create a balanced meal that you would enjoy. Pick a food from each food group and then write down the nutrients that each food gives you.

Table 4.9 **Now You Create a Balanced Meal! (example)**

Food Group	Your Food Choice	Nutrients Food Gives You
Grains	Multi-grain roll	Carbohydrates
Fruits	Oranges	Water, carbohydrates, vitamins
Vegetables	Spinach	Minerals, carbohydrates
Meat, Poultry, Fish, Dry Beans, Eggs, and Nuts	Baked chicken	Protein, vitamins, fat
Dairy	1% milk	Water, protein, carbohydrates, vitamins, fat

Fast-Food Frenzy

Background

Fat is an important part of our diets. It helps in the absorption and transport of fat-soluble vitamins, such as vitamins A, D, E, and K. Fat is the primary way energy is stored in the body, and fat can also make food taste good. In addition, components of fat are also involved in other important body functions such as maintaining healthy skin and hair.

The problem is that most Americans consume both too much fat and the wrong type of fat (namely, saturated fat and *trans* fat). This is thought to be one of the main reasons there are so many people who die of or are disabled by heart attacks in the United States. Every year, over half a million people die from heart disease in this country; heart disease is the leading cause of early death and disability in the United States. Studies have shown a strong relationship between high fat intake (especially saturated fat from animal sources, and *trans* fat from partially hydrogenated vegetable oils) and heart disease. The good news is that decreasing the intake of these fats helps reduce our risk of heart disease.

The Food Guide Pyramid is designed to help decrease daily fat intake to no more than 30 percent of total calories from fat. A diet low in fat, especially saturated and *trans* fats, may help maintain a healthy body weight as well as reduce the risk of heart disease. Therefore, it is important to identify the high-fat foods within each category of the Pyramid. Dairy foods, animal meats, and processed or fried foods tend to contain a lot more fat, especially the bad fats such as cholesterol, saturated fat, and *trans* fat (see "Fats: The Good Guys and the Bad Guys," lesson 6) than other foods in the pyramid.

However, within each of these food groups, there are lower-fat options from which to choose. Low-fat or nonfat milk, yogurt, and cheese are easy to find in any supermarket. Fish, poultry without skin, and dried beans provide protein without a lot of saturated fat. Foods found in the "fats, sweets, and oils" food group at the very top of the pyramid should be consumed in small quantities and relatively infrequently. Many foods that we call "junk" foods fit into this food group and tend to be very high in fat, sugar, and salt, but low in nutrients that help to decrease the risk for disease or infection.

The place to find out whether a food is relatively high or low in a nutrient is the % Daily Value column on the Nutrition Facts label on food packages. The % Daily Value for total fat and saturated fat are important. If the % Daily Value is 5 or less for an individual food, the food is considered low-fat (low in total fat and saturated fat). The more foods chosen that have a % Daily Value of 5 or less for total fat and saturated fat, the easier it is to eat a healthier daily diet. The overall daily goal should be to select foods that together do not exceed 100% of the Daily Value for total fat and saturated fat.

The % Daily Value is based on a diet of 2,000 calories per day.

How is % Daily Value for Fat Calculated?

Although all food labels provide %DV for nutrients, the following describes how the % Daily Value for one specific nutrient (fat) is calculated.

For a particular food, divide the number of grams of fat per serving by 65. Sixty-five (65) is used because it is recommended that a person eating a 2,000-calorie daily diet consume no more than 65 grams of fat each day.

For example: A serving of tuna salad has 14 grams of fat; $14 \div 65 = 22\%$. Therefore a serving of tuna salad contains 22% DV for fat for a person who eats 2,000 calories a day.

Estimated Teaching Time and Related Subject Areas

Estimated teaching time: 65 minutes

Related subject areas: language arts, math, science

Objectives

1. Students will be able to assess the fat content of their favorite fast-food meals.
2. Students will be able to design a low-fat, fast-food meal (≤34% Daily Value for fat).

Materials

1. Transparency #1, "Reading Food Labels"
2. Worksheet #1, "Adding Up the Fat"
3. Solutions to worksheet #1

Procedure

1. Ask the students to raise their hands if they like to eat at fast-food restaurants.
2. Have the students tell you their favorite fast-food eating places.
3. Explain that in today's lesson, students will have a chance to learn something about some of their favorite fast foods, especially how much fat they contain. Tell them that a lot of fast foods are high in total fat, saturated fat and *trans* fat. Since *trans* fat is not currently on the food label, students will concentrate on total fat for the activity.
4. Have each student write down all the foods that make up his or her favorite fast-food meal, including side orders like French fries, salads, drinks, or desserts, if they usually order them.
5. Review with students the concept of % Daily Value, discussed earlier. Display transparency #1, "Reading Food Labels." Ask students what they remember about the % Daily Value column.
6. Remind students that the % Daily Value lets them find out whether a food is high or low in a nutrient. Regarding fat, saturated fat, and cholesterol, if the % Daily Value is 5 or less for individual foods, then the food is considered low in those nutrients. The more foods chosen that have a % Daily Value of 5 or less for fat, the easier it is to eat a healthier daily diet.
7. The overall daily goal (for all the foods you eat in a day) should be to select foods that together do not exceed 100% of the Daily Value for fat. For a meal like lunch or dinner, a good goal may be to have a total % Daily Value for fat less than 34%. [34% is approximately a third of the daily 100% DV.]

Teacher/Student note: The use of 34% Daily Value for fat for a meal like lunch or dinner is simply an approximation of what someone might eat for lunch or dinner. It has been picked to help provide a standard for the class activity and is not a recommendation. Remind students that they need to focus on the overall recommendation that a person's total for a complete day be no more than 100% DV for fat.

8. Distribute the "Adding Up the Fat" worksheet and have each student determine the total % Daily Value for fat for his or her favorite fast-food meal. Students who can't find an item from their meal on the list should use the number of fat grams from an item most like the one they chose.

Most fast-food restaurants have nutrition information available to those who ask. Such information is also often available on the restaurants' home pages on the World Wide Web.

9. Explain to the students that a healthy lunch or dinner should not (on average) contain more than 34% DV for fat (both hidden in foods and added to foods), and slightly less would be even better.

   Also tell the students that although fast-food eating places are favorites of many young people, most fast foods are high in salt, saturated fat, and *trans* fat; and they are low in fiber. This is just the opposite of the diet recommended for staying healthy and lowering the risk of diseases, such as heart disease and cancer.

10. Ask the students how many of their fast-food meals contained less than 34% DV for fat. If any did, list the items from those meals on the board.

11. Have the students form pairs or small groups. Ask them to create a low-fat lunch (less than 34% DV for fat) that most of them would enjoy by selecting low-fat choices from the fast-food selections and/or "Alternative Sandwiches" list (found on "Adding Up the Fat"). Have students write down their choices on large sheets of paper, including each menu choice and what % DV for fat it contains.

12. Post the *healthier* menus and ask the groups to share their menus with the class. Encourage the students to think of these lower-fat items when they eat at a fast-food restaurant.

13. Stress that they should not be fearful of fat. It's OK to eat up to one small serving each day of high-fat foods (also known as "sometimes" foods). Moderation is the message. Choose foods that are low in saturated fat, *trans* fat, and cholesterol.

14. Follow-up: Have students create an advertisement that would appeal to others their age for a low-fat meal at a fast-food restaurant. This ad may be designed for a magazine or billboard (poster), television (skit, jingle), or radio (dialogue, jingle).

   Have students write a paragraph in their journal about five important things they have learned about fat.

Reading Food Labels

Reading food labels

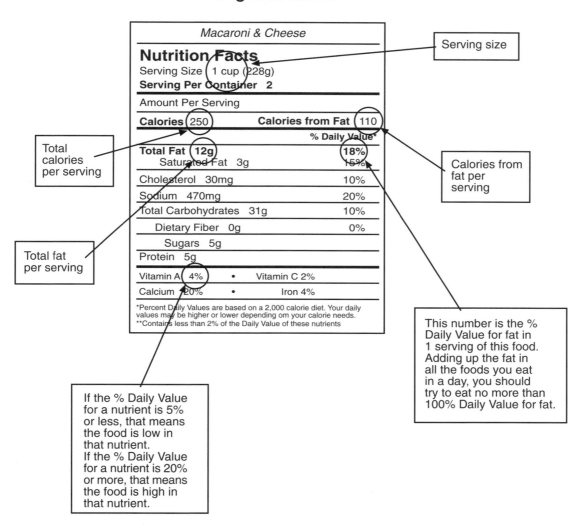

Macaroni & Cheese

Nutrition Facts
Serving Size 1 cup (228g)
Serving Per Container 2

Amount Per Serving

Calories 250   **Calories from Fat** 110

                                        % Daily Value*

Total Fat 12g   **18%**
   Saturated Fat 3g   15%

Cholesterol 30mg   10%

Sodium 470mg   20%

Total Carbohydrates 31g   10%

   Dietary Fiber 0g   0%

   Sugars 5g

Protein 5g

Vitamin A 4%   •   Vitamin C 2%

Calcium 20%   •   Iron 4%

*Percent Daily Values are based on a 2,000 calorie diet. Your daily
values may be higher or lower depending om your calorie needs.
**Contains less than 2% of the Daily Value of these nutrients

Serving size

Total calories per serving

Calories from fat per serving

Total fat per serving

This number is the % Daily Value for fat in 1 serving of this food. Adding up the fat in all the foods you eat in a day, you should try to eat no more than 100% Daily Value for fat.

If the % Daily Value for a nutrient is 5% or less, that means the food is low in that nutrient. If the % Daily Value for a nutrient is 20% or more, that means the food is high in that nutrient.

1 Adding Up the Fat

How much fat do the most common foods at your favorite fast-food restaurant contain? This activity will help you find out.

Directions

1. Look at the foods you chose for your favorite fast-food meal. Find those foods on the following lists. If one of your foods isn't here, find one that seems most like it.
2. In the right-hand column, find the % Daily Value for fat contained in one serving of that food. Circle these for each of the foods you choose.
3. Add up all the % Daily Values (%DV) for fat that you circled. Write the number in the answer box on page 2.
4. Decide whether the total is greater than, equal to, or less than 34%. Circle the correct choice in the answer box on page 2.

Table 5.1 % Daily Values of Fat for Fast Food

Hamburgers	Grams of Fat	%DV Fat	Pizza, Tacos, Chili	Grams of Fat	%DV Fat
Burger King Whopper	41	63	Wendy's Chili	9	14
Jack-in-the-Box Jumbo Jack	28	43	1/2 13" Thin 'n Crispy Pizza Hut Pizza Supreme	34	52
McDonald's Big Mac	33	51	Pizza Hut Standard, cheese 1/2 13"	38	58
Wendy's Old-Fashioned Cheeseburger	14	22	Jack-in-the-Box Taco	26	40
McDonald's Quarter Pounder	22	34	Taco Bell Bean Burrito	12	18
McDonald's Quarter Pounder with cheese	31	48	Taco Bell Beef Burrito	21	32
			Taco Bell Beefy Tostada	15	23
Burger King Double Whopper with cheese	60	92	Taco Bell Enchirito	21	32
Burger King Whopper Junior	20	31	Taco Bell Tacos	8	12
Wendy's Double with cheese	48	74	**Other Fast Food Items**		
McDonald's Plain Hamburger	11	17	French fries, regular	11	17
Fish			Onion rings	16	25
			Shakes, regular	9	14
Long John Silver's	27	42	Roll with butter	7	11
Arthur Treacher's Original	27	42	Salad bar	5-20	8-13
McDonald's Filet-O-Fish	25	38	Coleslaw	11	17
Burger King Whaler	34	52			

Sandwiches	Grams of Fat	%DV Fat
Roy Roger's Roast Beef Sandwich ...	12	18
Burger King Chopped Beef Steak Sandwich	13	20
Hardee's Roast Beef Sandwich	17	26
Arby's Roast Beef Sandwich	15	23
Arby's Roast Beef with cheese	22	34
Arby's Super Roast Beef	28	43
Arby's Turkey Deluxe	24	37

Desserts

	Grams of Fat	%DV Fat
McDonald's Apple or Cherry Pie	14	22
McDonald's Cookies	11	17
McDonald's Hot Fudge Sundae ...	11	17
Dairy Queen Banana Split...........	15	23
Dairy Queen Freeze	13	20
Dairy Queen Hot Fudge Brownie Delight	22	34
Dairy Queen Ice Cream Sandwich	14	22
Jack-in-the Box Apple Turnover ...	24	37

Drinks

	Grams of Fat	%DV Fat
100% Fruit Juices	0	0
1% milk (8 oz.)	2.4	5

Chicken	Grams of Fat	%DV Fat
Kentucky Fried Chicken Snack Box	21	32
Arthur Treacher's Original Chicken	23	35
McDonald's McNuggets	19	29
Kentucky Fried Chicken Extra Crispy Dinners	45	70

Alternative Sandwiches

	Grams of Fat	%DV Fat
Low-fat chicken salad.................	15	23
Swiss cheese with mustard	16	25
Chicken breast	12	18
Plain roast beef	22	34
Tuna salad	14	22
Eggplant parmesan sub with low-fat cheese	15	23

Combination Dishes

	Grams of Fat	%DV Fat
Beef teriyaki with rice and vegetables	11	22
Spaghetti with meat sauce	12	18
Spaghetti with tomato sauce........	9	14
Meatless chili	7	11
Macaroni and cheese	14	22
Lasagna with meat	24	37

Center for Science in the the Public Interest, *Nutrition Action Health Letter; Diet for the Young at Heart*, Best Foods; *Food Values*, Pennington and Church

Table 5.2 Answers

1. What is the total % Daily Value (DV) for fat? _____

2. Into which of the following categories does your answer to question #1 belong? (circle one)

   Greater than 34%
   Equal to 34%
   Less than 34%

Calculation of % Daily Value for fat is based on a person needing 2,000 calories per day.

Solutions

Worksheet 1   Adding Up the Fat

How much fat do the most common foods at your favorite fast-food restaurant contain? This activity will help you find out.

Directions

1. Look at the foods you chose for your favorite fast-food meal. Find those foods on the following lists. If one of your foods isn't here, find one that seems most like it.
2. In the right-hand column, find the % Daily Value for fat contained in one serving of that food. Circle these for each of the foods you chose.
3. Add up all the % Daily Values (%DV) for fat that you circled. Write the number in the answer box on page 2.
4. Decide whether the total is greater than, equal to, or less than 34%. Circle the correct choice in the answer box on page 2.

Table 5.3   % Daily Values of Fat for Fast Food

Hamburgers	Grams of Fat	%DV Fat
Burger King Whopper	41	63
Jack-in-the-Box Jumbo Jack	28	43
McDonald's Big Mac	33	51
Wendy's Old-Fashioned Cheeseburger	14	22
McDonald's Quarter Pounder	22	34
McDonald's Quarter Pounder with cheese	31	48
Burger King Double Whopper with cheese	60	92
Burger King Whopper Junior	20	31
Wendy's Double with cheese	48	74
McDonald's Plain Hamburger	11	17

Fish		
Long John Silver's	27	42
Arthur Treacher's Original	27	42
McDonald's Filet-O-Fish	25	38
Burger King Whaler	34	52

Pizza, Tacos, Chili	Grams of Fat	%DV Fat
Wendy's Chili	9	14
1/2 13" Thin 'n Crispy Pizza Hut Pizza Supreme	34	52
Pizza Hut Standard, cheese 1/2 13"	38	58
Jack-in-the-Box Taco	26	40
Taco Bell Bean Burrito	12	18
Taco Bell Beef Burrito	21	32
Taco Bell Beefy Tostada	15	23
Taco Bell Enchirito	21	32
Taco Bell Tacos	8	12

Other Fast Food Items		
French fries, regular	11	17
Onion rings	16	25
Shakes, regular	9	14
Roll with butter	7	11
Salad bar	5-20	8-13
Coleslaw	11	17

Sandwiches	Grams of Fat	%DV Fat
Roy Roger's Roast Beef Sandwich ...	12	18
Burger King Chopped Beef Steak Sandwich	13	20
Hardee's Roast Beef Sandwich	17	26
Arby's Roast Beef Sandwich	15	23
Arby's Roast Beef with cheese	22	34
Arby's Super Roast Beef	28	43
Arby's Turkey Deluxe	24	37

Desserts

	Grams of Fat	%DV Fat
McDonald's Apple or Cherry Pie	14	22
McDonald's Cookies	11	17
McDonald's Hot Fudge Sundae ...	11	17
Dairy Queen Banana Split...........	15	23
Dairy Queen Freeze	13	20
Dairy Queen Hot Fudge Brownie Delight	22	34
Dairy Queen Ice Cream Sandwich	14	22
Jack-in-the Box Apple Turnover ...	24	37

Drinks

	Grams of Fat	%DV Fat
100% Fruit Juices	0	0
1% milk (8 oz.)	2.4	5

Chicken	Grams of Fat	%DV Fat
Kentucky Fried Chicken Snack Box	21	32
Arthur Treacher's Original Chicken	23	35
McDonald's McNuggets	19	29
Kentucky Fried Chicken Extra Crispy Dinners	45	70

Alternative Sandwiches

	Grams of Fat	%DV Fat
Low-fat chicken salad..................	15	23
Swiss cheese with mustard	16	25
Chicken breast	12	18
Plain roast beef	22	34
Tuna salad	14	22
Eggplant parmesan sub with low-fat cheese	15	23

Combination Dishes

	Grams of Fat	%DV Fat
Beef teriyaki with rice and vegetables	11	22
Spaghetti with meat sauce	12	18
Spaghetti with tomato sauce........	9	14
Meatless chili	7	11
Macaroni and cheese	14	22
Lasagna with meat	24	37

Center for Science in the the Public Interest, *Nutrition Action Health Letter; Diet for the Young at Heart*, Best Foods; *Food Values*, Pennington and Church

Table 5.4 Answers

1. What is the total % Daily Value (DV) for fat? _____ **52** _____

2. Into which of the following categories does
   your answer to question #1 belong? (circle one)   Greater than 34%
                                                        Equal to 34 %
                                                        Less than 34 %

Calculation of % Daily Value for fat is based on a person needing 2,000 calories per day.

Snack Attack

Background

There are "sometimes" foods and there are "everyday" foods, but there are no "bad" foods that should never be eaten. However, many Americans tend to eat too many foods high in saturated and *trans* fats, salt, and refined sugar. (Did you know that one 12-ounce can of regular soda contains about 10 teaspoons of sugar?) Because snack foods tend to have a lot of these, they often appear at the top of the Food Guide Pyramid: ideally one should eat only limited amounts of these kinds of foods ("sometimes" foods), and should eat more of the nutrient-rich foods at the base of the pyramid ("everyday" foods).

The purpose of this lesson is to help students make better snack choices by recognizing sources of fat—especially sources of saturated and *trans* fats. It is important to remember that most saturated fat comes from animal sources (including beef, chicken, pork, and dairy products). The few exceptions are coconut oil and palm oil, which are also rich in saturated fat. *Trans* fat comes from hydrogenation of vegetable oils. This process turns the oils into solid fats.

Fats: The Good Guys and the Bad Guys

The good guys—monounsaturated and polyunsaturated fats. These fats are from plant sources or fish, and are liquid at room temperature. Substituting these types of fats for saturated and trans fats may decrease the risk of heart disease. Examples of foods high in monounsaturated fats include olive, canola, and peanut oils. Nuts, soybean oil, corn oil, and cottonseed oil are rich in polyunsaturated fats. Fatty ocean fish contain a special type of polyunsaturated fat.

However, remember that moderation is the key to healthy eating; and that principal holds true with the intake of monounsaturated and polyunsaturated fats.

The bad guys—saturated fat, *trans* fat, and cholesterol. Saturated fat is mainly from animals. Examples include high-fat dairy products (like whole milk, cream, butter, regular-fat ice cream), skin of poultry, palm oil, coconut oil, and lard. Minimize the intake of these foods.

Trans fat is made when the process of hydrogenation changes the polyunsaturated fat that is normally present in the vegetable oils into solid fat. Examples of *trans* fat include partially hydrogenated vegetable oils (e.g., partially hydrogenated soybean or sunflower seed oil). Watch out for the words "hydrogenated vegetable oils" in labels of hard margarines, snacks, commercially fried foods, and cookies. Hydrogenated oils are rich sources of *trans* fat. Research has shown an increase of heart disease risk with increased consumption of saturated or trans fat.

Foods high in dietary cholesterol tend to raise blood cholesterol. Examples include egg yolks, liver and organ meats, and dairy fat. Minimize the intake of these foods.

Reading food labels is an effective way to compare the fat and nutrient content of various snack foods. The place to find out whether a food is relatively high or low in a nutrient is the % Daily Value column on the Nutrition Facts label. (Total fat, saturated fat, and cholesterol are currently listed on food labels. The FDA is considering listing *trans* fat as well.) The % Daily Value for fat is important. If, for individual foods, the % Daily Value is 5 or less, the food is considered low fat. The more foods chosen that have a % Daily Value of 5 or less for fat, the easier it is to eat a healthier daily diet. The overall daily goal should be to select foods that together do not exceed 100% of the Daily Value for fat. (To learn how to calculate % Daily Value for fat, see "How is % Daily Value for Fat Calculated?" in lesson 5, page 60. The % Daily Value is based on a diet of 2,000 calories per day.)

Estimated Teaching Time and Related Subject Areas

Estimated teaching time: 1 hour, 30 minutes

Related subject areas: science, math, art

Objectives

1. Students will describe the importance of selecting healthful snacks.
2. Students will analyze food labels to locate information on caloric and fat content.

Materials

1. Transparency #1, "Snack Time"
2. Transparency #2, "Reading Food Labels"
3. Worksheet #1, "Be Fat Wise"
4. Worksheet #2, "Snacking the Fast-Food Way"
5. Solutions to worksheet #1
6. Solutions to worksheet #2
7. Solutions to "% Daily Value Snack Choices Exercise"
8. A variety of empty snack food packages. (You may have students bring these in.)

Motivation

1. Have students make a list of their 10 favorite snack foods or beverages.
2. Show the "Snack Time" transparency. Have students identify the pyramid group in which each snack belongs. Fill in snack names in the appropriate space on the pyramid.
3. Discussion questions

   Question 1: Into which group were most of their snacks placed?

   Question 2: Were most of their snack choices low in fat, salt, and/or sugar?
4. Explain to students that foods in each food group may move to the top of the pyramid if they have excess fat and sugar. For example, a cup cake is made from grains (flour), but because of its high amounts of fat and refined sugar, it belongs at the top of the pyramid.

Procedure

1. Discuss the importance of selecting on a regular basis foods that are low in saturated and *trans* fats. Note that high-fat snacks, *regardless of the type of fat,* are usually high-calorie foods that, when used in excess, may promote excessive weight gain. The body stores fat as an energy reserve, and can do so in almost unlimited amounts. However, eating high-fat snacks ("sometimes food") once in a while is fine.

2. Have students complete the "Be Fat Wise" worksheet individually or in pairs. Review the answers. (See solutions.)

3. Distribute the "Snacking the Fast-Food Way" worksheet. Have students work in pairs to complete the activities described. Review the answers. (See solutions.)

4. Give each pair of students the number of grams of fat in the selections from one of the sets (see "Snacking the Fast Food Way" Solutions). Have the students make bar graphs to compare the fat content. Post the graphs as a visual reminder of the comparisons.

5. Show the "Reading Food Labels" transparency and explain the labeled information. Explain that reading the labels is the way to determine the fat content of the foods we eat.

6. Distribute food packages representing popular snack foods. Have students locate and record the calories per serving, the amount of fat grams per serving, the calories from fat per serving, and the percent of Daily Value (% DV) for fat as listed on the food label. Also look at the ingredients list and identify foods that contain *trans* fat (partially hydrogenated oils).

7. Determine which snacks together would add up to 100% of the recommended daily maximum of fat (add the percents of daily value to equal 100%). It may take only two to four snacks, depending on their fat content. Explain that just those snacks alone would contain a person's daily maximum allowance of fat (100% of the Daily Value). (See solutions.)

   The % Daily Value (based on a 2,000-calorie diet) can help you follow nutrition experts' advice not to eat more than 30% of your calories from fat. All you need to do is add up the % DV for fat in all the foods you eat in a day. Your goal is to eat no more than 100% DV for fat.

8. Explain to students that high-fat snacks can be eaten once in a while and should be considered "sometimes foods." On a regular basis, they should choose more foods that are lower in fat.

Extension Activities

1. Have students create a Snack Food Pyramid which shows low-fat choices in each of the following food groups.

Food group	Examples
Bread, cereal, rice, and pasta	whole wheat pretzels
Vegetable	carrots
Fruit	apple
Milk, yogurt, and cheese	low-fat yogurt
Meat, poultry, fish, dry beans, eggs, and nuts	bean spread

2. Have students design a label for a low-fat snack food that would appeal to their peers.

3. Research the link between dietary fat and heart disease.

4. Have students identify snack foods that are high in refined sugar (e.g., cup cakes, candy bars, soda) or salt (e.g., chips, cheese curls). Have them think of healthier alternatives (e.g., four favorite fruits cut up and put in a bowl, toasted pita bread strips or tortilla chips made with no hydrogenated fats dipped in mild salsa).

Snack Time

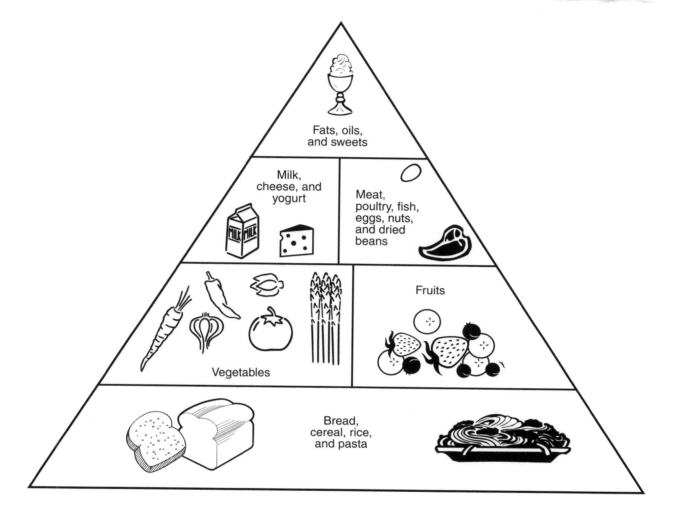

Fats, oils,
and sweets

Milk,
cheese, and
yogurt

Meat,
poultry, fish,
eggs, nuts,
and dried
beans

Vegetables

Fruits

Bread,
cereal, rice,
and pasta

2 Reading Food Labels

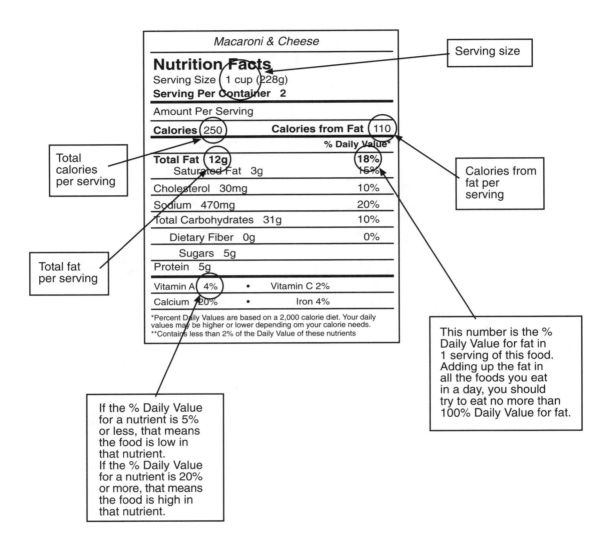

Serving size

Total calories per serving

Calories from fat per serving

Total fat per serving

Macaroni & Cheese

Nutrition Facts
Serving Size 1 cup (228g)
Serving Per Container 2

Amount Per Serving

Calories 250   **Calories from Fat** 110

                                                    % Daily Value*

Total Fat 12g   **18%**
   Saturated Fat 3g   15%

Cholesterol 30mg   10%

Sodium 470mg   20%

Total Carbohydrates 31g   10%

   Dietary Fiber 0g   0%

   Sugars 5g

Protein 5g

Vitamin A 4%   •   Vitamin C 2%

Calcium 20%   •   Iron 4%

*Percent Daily Values are based on a 2,000 calorie diet. Your daily values may be higher or lower depending om your calorie needs.
**Contains less than 2% of the Daily Value of these nutrients

This number is the % Daily Value for fat in 1 serving of this food. Adding up the fat in all the foods you eat in a day, you should try to eat no more than 100% Daily Value for fat.

If the % Daily Value for a nutrient is 5% or less, that means the food is low in that nutrient.
If the % Daily Value for a nutrient is 20% or more, that means the food is high in that nutrient.

Be Fat Wise

Directions

Put the foods below in each line in order to show if they are high-fat, moderate-fat, or low-fat snack foods.

Group 1: ice cream, low-fat frozen yogurt, sherbet

Group 2: angel food cake, apple pie, poptart

Group 3: bagel, doughnut, low-fat muffin

Group 4: flour tortilla, tortilla chips, corn tortilla

Group 5: potato chips, pretzels, saltine crackers

Group 6: bologna, lean red meat, roast turkey

Table 6.1 Be Fat Wise

	High-Fat "Sometimes Foods"	Moderate-Fat	Low-Fat
Example	French fries	baked potato with butter	baked potato with low-fat yogurt
Group 1			
Group 2			
Group 3			
Group 4			
Group 5			
Group 6			

Snacking the Fast-Food Way

Directions

For each set below, place an (X) in the box next to the food that contains more fat.

Table 6.2   Snacking the Fast-Food Way

❏ 1 cheeseburger ❏ 2 slices of cheese pizza	❏ 1 slice apple pie with 1/2 cup of ice cream ❏ apple with 1 cup low-fat yogurt
❏ 1 doughnut ❏ 1 bagel	❏ 1 oz. pretzels ❏ 1 oz. potato chips
❏ 1 taco ❏ 3 oz. roasted chicken	❏ 1 cup 1% chocolate milk ❏ 1 chocolate milkshake
❏ Wendy's baked potato ❏ Wendy's fries	❏ Burger King Whopper with cheese ❏ Burger King Chicken Tenders
❏ KFC mashed potatoes ❏ KFC fries	❏ KFC baked beans ❏ KFC buttermilk biscuit
❏ McDonald's Filet O'Fish ❏ McDonald's Chunky Chicken Salad w/ Vinaigrette dressing	❏ McDonald's English Muffin ❏ McDonald's Sausage Muffin

Solutions

Worksheet 1   Be Fat Wise

Directions

Put the foods below in each line in order to show if they are high-fat, moderate-fat, or low-fat snack foods.

Table 6.3   Be Fat Wise Solutions

	High-Fat "Sometimes Foods"	Moderate-Fat	Low-Fat
Group 1	ice cream	low-fat frozen yogurt	sherbet
Group 2	apple pie	poptart	angel food cake
Group 3	doughnut	muffin	bagel
Group 4	tortilla chips	flour tortilla	corn tortilla
Group 5	potato chips	saltine crackers	pretzels
Group 6	bologna	lean red meat	roast turkey

Solutions

Worksheet 2   Snacking the Fast-Food Way

An (X) is next to the food that contains more fat in each set below. The number of grams of fat for each food is also given.

Table 6.4   Snacking the Fast-Food Way Solutions

Grams of fat in each selection:

☒ (20) 1 cheeseburger ☐ (5) 2 slices of cheese pizza	☒ (20) 1 slice apple pie with 1/2 cup of ice cream ☐ (4) apple with 1 cup low-fat yogurt
☒ (12) 1 doughnut ☐ (1) 1 bagel	☐ (2) 1 oz. pretzels ☒ (9) 1 oz. potato chips
☒ (21) 1 taco ☐ (3) 3 oz. roasted chicken	☐ (3) 1 cup 1% chocolate milk ☒ (11) 1 chocolate milkshake
☐ (1) Wendy's baked potato ☒ (15) Wendy's fries	☒ (48) Burger King Whopper with cheese ☐ (10) Burger King Chicken Tenders
☐ (1) KFC mashed potatoes ☒ (13) KFC fries	☐ (1) KFC baked beans ☒ (14) KFC buttermilk biscuit
☒ (26) McDonald's Filet O'Fish ☐ (9) McDonald's Chunky Chicken Salad w/ Vinaigrette dressing	☐ (6) McDonald's English Muffin ☒ (31) McDonald's Sausage Muffin

Solutions

% Daily Value Snack Choices Exercise

Example of snack choices totaling 100% Daily Value for fat

Snack Foods	% Daily Value (DV) for Fat
Skim milk	0%
Fruit salad	0%
Macaroni and cheese (2 servings)	52%
Frosted doughnuts	35%
Tuna (water-packed)	8%
Orange juice	0%
Spinach	0%
Reduced-fat cheese	5%
Total	100%

The Safe Workout: Snacking's Just Fine, If You Choose the Right Kind

Background

This lesson helps teach students the importance of movement and eating well for a healthy body. The lesson includes the five parts of a safe workout, the different parts of fitness, and a nutrition concept (healthful snacks). The exciting part of this lesson is that the students will be moving while they are learning!

Snacks can be an important part of a child's diet. For students, snacks (if chosen wisely) can help provide the calories and nutrients that they need for growth, development, and physical activity.

Students should learn how to choose healthier snacks. Often, they choose highly processed snacks that are high in salt, refined sugar, saturated fat, and *trans* fat. These snacks are high in calories and low in important nutrients (like vitamins and minerals) and are said to be filled with "empty" calories—calories that are not accompanied by healthful nutrients. Snacks like fruit, low-fat yogurt, and whole wheat bread, on the other hand, are "nutrient-dense"—they contain calories that are accompanied by vitamins and minerals. However, children on average are not getting enough fruits and vegetables (5-A-Day). They need to understand the importance of choosing nutrient-dense snacks rather than snacks filled with empty calories. Recommend fruits, vegetables, and whole grain products as snacks.

Overview

This lesson reviews the different parts of a safe workout and includes an endurance fitness activity where students "shop" for healthful snacks.

Estimated Teaching Time and Related Subject Area

Estimated teaching time: 1 hour

Related subject area: health

Objectives

1. Students will discuss and demonstrate each component of a safe workout.
2. Students will understand the importance of movement/physical activity as part of a healthy lifestyle.
3. Students will understand the benefits of choosing healthful snacks over less healthful snacks.

Materials

1. Pictures of various snack foods
2. Food Guide Pyramid poster
3. Stretching and Strength Fitness diagrams (see appendix, pp. 453-459)
4. Portable tape deck/radio (optional)

Procedure

Part I: Vocabulary Terms Review

Warm-up: the first part of the safe workout, in which slow movements get the body ready for stretching and the fitness activity

Stretch: the part of the safe workout in which you do exercises that improve flexibility fitness and get the body ready for fitness activity

Fitness activity: the part of the safe workout in which strength and endurance fitness exercises are performed

Cool-down: the part of the safe workout in which your body slows down and recovers from the fitness activity

Cool-down stretch: the last part of the safe workout, in which you do exercises that improve flexibility fitness

Pacing: maintaining a comfortable speed so that you can perform your exercise over an extended period of time

Flexibility fitness: the part of fitness that stretches the muscles and areas around the muscles to get your body ready for action; ability to bend

Strength fitness: the part of fitness that gets your muscles stronger and healthier

Endurance fitness: the part of fitness that helps improve the heart muscle, lungs, and blood vessels and helps maintain weight

Part II: Pre-Warm-Up Introduction

1. Ask students: What is a snack? Should we eat snacks?
2. Discuss with students what they eat for snacks.
3. Ask students what they think the phrase "Snacking is just fine, if you choose the right kind" means.
4. Ask students, "Where in the Food Guide Pyramid do you find the healthful kinds of snacks?" (Possible answers: fruits and vegetables, whole grains, low-fat dairy.)
5. Discuss with students why fruits, vegetables, whole grains, and low-fat dairy foods are the right kind of snacks. (They contain healthful nutrients, like vitamins and minerals, that our bodies need.)
6. Have students name snacks from each of the following groups:

   Grains: bagels, whole wheat toast, whole wheat/low-fat crackers, rice cakes, pancakes

   Fruits: apples, oranges, grapes, kiwi, pears, 100% apple juice, raisins

   Vegetables: carrots, salad, broccoli, cauliflower, celery, cucumber slices

   Dairy (low-fat choices): skim milk, 1% milk, 1% chocolate milk, low-fat yogurt, low-fat frozen yogurt

Part III: Components of the Safe Workout

Place students into groups represented by the food groups of the Food Guide Pyramid (i.e., grain group, fruit group, etc.). Remind students that eating right and keeping their bodies moving (getting exercise) are equally important and together help keep them healthy and energized.

The following description covers all five areas of the safe workout, including the fitness activity—a movement game that involves choosing healthful snacks.

1. The warm-up (1-2 minutes)
2. The stretch (1-2 minutes)
3. The fitness activity (15-20 minutes)
4. The cool-down (1 minute)
5. The cool-down stretch (1 minute)
6. Stay healthy corner (4-5 minutes)

1. The Warm-Up: 1-2 Minutes

Music may be played during warm-up (optional).

What to Emphasize

- Car analogy: your body is like a cold car—warm it up and then move it!
- If you do not warm up, you are more likely to get injured.
- You should always warm up before exercising, even when you are at home.
- Always do the movements very slowly to warm up.
- For example, for a bike ride, warm up by riding slowly at first.
- Likewise, when throwing a ball, throw slowly at first.

Examples of Student Warm-Up Formations

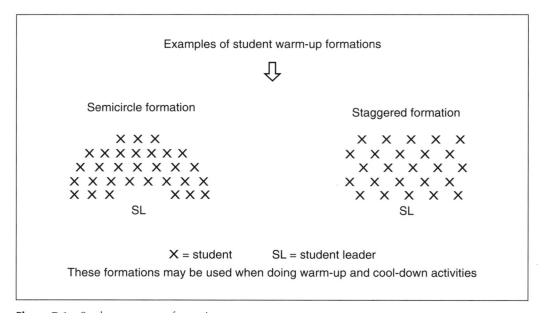

Figure 7.1 Student warm-up formations.

Semicircle Formation

1. Students should establish and maintain a safe distance between those students who are in front of, in back of, and on either side of themselves.
2. There should be enough room between students so that they will be able to do all stretches and exercises without fear of inadvertently hitting or being hit by another student.
3. Students should stand so they are facing the teacher and/or group leader. They should be spaced so there is not another student directly in front of them.

Staggered Formation

1. Have a group of five students form a row with enough space so that they cannot touch each other if their arms are extended at shoulder height. Five more students will form a second row behind row one. Students in the second row should stand behind and between the two students in the row in front of them and, like those in the first row, should make sure that there is enough space between them (and between them and students in front of them). Continue to put students in rows until all have been placed.

2. Students should stand so that they are facing (and can see) the teacher and/or student leader who will be in front of the room.

2. The Stretch: 1-2 Minutes

Examples of Student Stretches

Have students perform stretches as they appear in the diagrams in the appendix. One student or a small group of students can help demonstrate the stretches for the class.

What to Emphasize

- Stretching improves flexibility fitness.
- Activities such as riding a bike or doing push-ups do not improve flexibility.
- Even if you aren't going to be doing a fitness activity, stretch at home while watching TV or when doing nothing in particular.
- Hold stretches for 10 or more seconds.
- Use slow movements; don't bounce.

3. The Endurance Activity: 15-20 Minutes

What to Emphasize

- Pace, don't race.
- Getting fit should be fun.

Endurance Activity Game

Eat Well & *Keep Moving*: Choosing Healthful Snacks

a. Equipment needed
  1. A variety of snack pictures from the different food groups
  2. Five hula hoops or boxes (representing a refrigerator/plate)
  3. Music to move to (optional)

b. Introduction

  Explain to students, "The purpose of the game is to determine if each of you knows how to choose healthful snacks. We are also playing this game so that we can become more fit. We shall pace ourselves so that we can do an activity for a certain length of time without becoming tired, which will help us become stronger."

c. Procedure
  1. Have class form five groups. Each group could be named after a food group, e.g., the grain group. The teacher should represent the tip of the Pyramid: fats, oils, and sweets.
  2. Ask each group to form a line (see "Classroom Line Formation Options").
  3. Explain and demonstrate the paths the students will take so there is no confusion, and so that students can perform their tasks safely.
  4. A cone or a distinguishable line on the floor can mark the place where the first person in each line can stand. The second person in the line moves to this place after the first student has left it.
  5. Place a hula hoop to the right of each line of students (refer to the Line Formation diagram). This hula hoop can be called a plate or a refrigerator. Each student will place the food that he/she has collected in this area and then jog to the back of his/her food group line.
  6. Begin by asking all students who are first in line to take a step forward. You will now walk this group through the course that you would like them to take while pointing out the following:
     a) "The area inside the basketball key has pictures of food all over the floor and is called the grocery store. Each student will go shopping for a healthful snack. The first person in each group will jog in a straight path until s/he gets to the grocery store area. Once there, select a snack for your group, pick it up, and jog back to the area we are calling the plate/refrigerator (hula hoop) and deposit the food item in it. You will then jog to the back of your line and jog in place until every member of every group has completed this task."
     b) Remind students that this is not a race or a competition between groups. When the first student in each line is going through this, coach them by reminding them to come back on their path so that they can safely jog to their plate/refrigerator.

    c) Tell students to "pace, don't race," so they can continue jogging until each member of their group has gone shopping and brought back a snack item. Remind the next people in line to wait until the jogger has arrived at the end of the line before starting out, so that the activity can be done safely.

    d) After the first group of students has walked through the course and has moved to the back of the line, ask if there are any questions. If there are no questions, tell the students that they are about to begin with the set of students who are now first in line.

7. This activity will begin with the teacher saying, "Let's go shopping for snacks!" The entire class will jog lightly in place until the last student in each food group has had a turn and has taken a place at the end of the line.

8. Once all have completed the activity, tell the students it is time for the cool-down. Ask students to walk around the gymnasium, cafeteria, or community room three times, with everyone moving in the same direction.

4. The Cool-Down: 1 Minute

What to Emphasize

- Move slowly.
- Remember to cool down after exercising at home too.

5. The Cool-Down Stretch: 1 Minute

What to Emphasize

- Stretching improves flexibility fitness.
- Activities such as riding a bike or doing push-ups do not improve flexibility.
- Even if you aren't going to be doing a fitness activity, stretch at home while watching TV or when doing nothing in particular.
- Hold stretches for 10 or more seconds.
- Use slow movements; don't bounce.

6. The Stay Healthy Corner: 4-5 Minutes

During this time a nutrition concept related to the fitness activity will be introduced.

Choosing Healthier Snacks

1. Tell the students that the class will now look at the snack choices each group made.

2. Ask for volunteers from each group to share one or two of the snacks their group chose. Review students' choices and remind them that a healthful snack is one that is not highly processed, is low in saturated and *trans* fats, and is high in vitamins and minerals.

Classroom Line Formation Options

The best option depends on the layout of the classroom. See p. 89.

Gym line formation
for shopping fitness activities

[X = one student, □ = teacher (fats, oils, and sweets)]

The purpose of the game is to determine if each student in a group knows which food items from the Food Guide Pyramid fit into their food group. We are also playing this game so that we can become fit and learn how to pace ourselves so that we can make our bodies stronger and able to do an activity for a certain length of time without becoming tired.

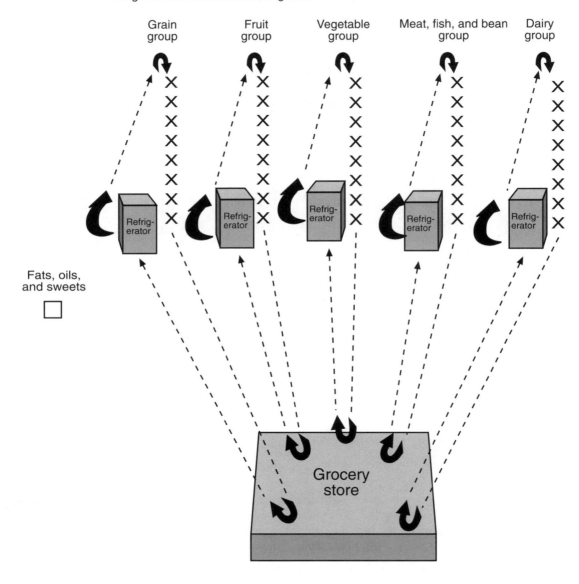

Classroom line formation options

The best option depends on the layout of the classroom

Option #1

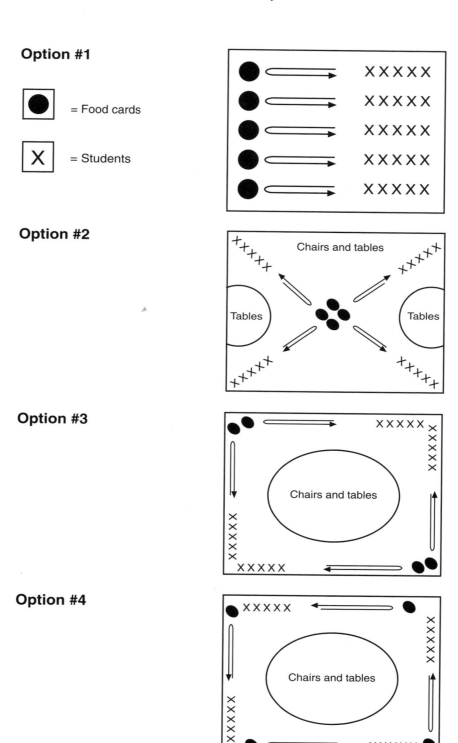

= Food cards

= Students

Option #2

Option #3

Option #4

Prime-Time Smartness

Background

During the late 1980s and early 1990s, 26% of all children watched over four hours of TV a day. Essentially, TV watching for many children has become a full-time job! On average, youth spend more time watching television each year than they spend in school. This tendency toward an inactive or sedentary lifestyle is a contributing factor to youths' being overweight. The more television a child watches, the more likely he or she will be overweight. The increase in television viewing has also been associated with elevated cholesterol levels and poor cardiovascular fitness in youth. Young people should be encouraged to consider healthy alternatives to television viewing, particularly choices that involve more physical activity.

Estimated Teaching Time and Related Subject Areas

Estimated teaching time: 1 hour, 30 minutes

Related subject areas: reading, math

Objectives

1. Students will identify a television program(s) they will not view in order to participate in an alternative activity.
2. Students will create a list of alternative activities to consider in place of watching television.

Materials

1. Envelopes containing "Dear Student" letter and "Pledge"—one per student
2. Small white envelopes for signed copy of the pledge—one per student
3. Worksheet #1, "My Favorite Prime-Time Shows"
4. Packet of "Prime-Time Smartness Challenge" materials (one for each student who wants to take the challenge):

   "Hello Again"

   "The Star Page"

   "The Questions Page"
5. Certificate of Congratulations for students who take the challenge
6. *Freeze My TV* program summary

Procedure

Part I: Motivation

1. Begin by telling class that the office has delivered special letters addressed to "Students Only." The teacher should also receive a letter marked "Teacher Only." (Pass out a letter to each child, with address similar to following example.)

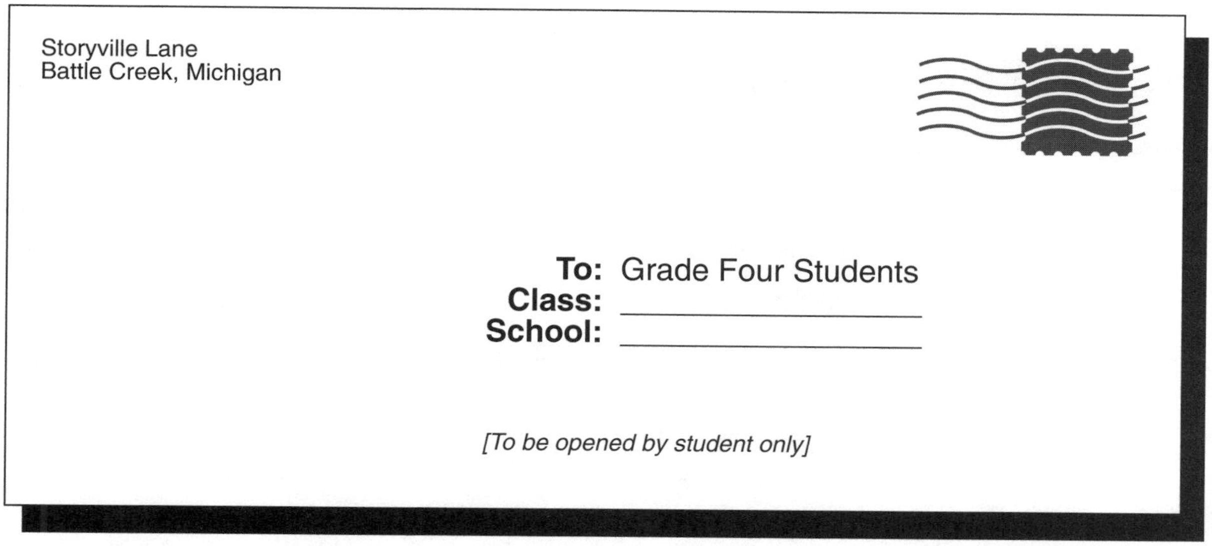

Storyville Lane
Battle Creek, Michigan

To: Grade Four Students
Class: _____
School: _____

[To be opened by student only]

Figure 8.1 "Students Only" address example.

Option: If your school can afford the expense (approximately $10.00 total for postage), have the letters mailed to each student in the class.

2. Provide time for the class to open the letters and read the pages quietly. Encourage students who need assistance to work in pairs.

3. Pretend to open the "teacher only" letter, then tell students that they have been asked to create a list of things that could be done at home in "prime-time" hours. (Write the words "prime time" on the board.)

Part II: Development

1. Ask students to tell the meaning of "prime time" as it relates to television viewing. (Note: Prime time refers to the period of the day during which most programs on television record their highest viewing audience.)

2. Have students identify some favorite shows that they watch between 4 p.m. and 9 p.m.

3. Conduct a class poll to determine the class's favorite shows: first choice, second choice, and third choice.

Program	Show #1	Show #2	Show #3
A. The Simpsons	18	15	1
B. Pokémon	10	14	10
C. Batman	6	5	23

Figure 8.2 Sample: students identify favorite shows (first, second, and third choice).

4. Ask students to study the chart to determine which program would probably be easiest for the class to "pass up." (In the example above, Batman was chosen as a third choice by more students, so it would probably be the easiest not to watch.)

5. Ask students to think of activities in which they could participate when not watching television. (As the list is brainstormed, record answers on the board. List at least 7 to 10 activities.)

Sample alternatives to TV: Read a book, write a poem, play a game with brother/sister, help a little brother/sister, play basketball, dance, walk to the store, help with chores.

Part III: Application

1. Have students review and discuss the list to determine if activities are safe (not dangerous) to do.

2. Guide students in reviewing the list again to determine which activities involve the greatest level of physical activity.

3. Guide them in coding the list as follows:

   (+) = some physical activity (e.g., dancing, stretching, playing ball)

   (–) = very little physical activity (e.g., reading, playing a board game)

   Have students cite the benefits of choosing activities that involve physical activity.

   Sample Benefits:
   - Exercises the muscles.
   - Exercises the heart.

4. Distribute "My Favorite Prime-Time Shows." Have students write in their three favorite television programs for each day. Ask them to circle one for each day that they would agree to pass up if they were to take "The Prime-Time Smartness Challenge" (see extension).

Part IV: Summary and Extension

1. Explain the "Prime-Time Smartness Challenge" to students. Record names of students who agree to participate. Distribute packet of materials.

   The Challenge does not have to be limited to students who watch TV. If a student does not watch any TV, he or she can still participate in the daily activities of the Challenge. Where appropriate, instead of substituting for television time, the student may substitute physically active time for physically inactive time. For example, instead of sitting and listening to music, the student could dance to the music.

2. Create a bulletin board titled "Winner's Circle." Display pictures of students who participate in the "Prime-Time Challenge." Add the "Certificates of Congratulations" of those students who return their materials to the teacher.

3. Make a bar graph with the class to show the numbers of students who give up 30 minutes of television each day for the week. Each morning, have one of the students fill in the bar for the previous day.

4. Make a pie chart of an average day (24 hours). Have the students estimate and display the number of hours each day they do the following activities:

Sleep	Do homework
Eat	Bathe/dress/brush teeth, etc.
Spend in school	Other activities
Play	

5. Explain the *Freeze My TV* promotion to students (summary provided; also see lesson 25). Tell them it will be another TV-related activity they will participate in.

Dear Student:

How would you like to be smarter in just 5 days? Yes, that's right! You can be smarter than you are now in just 5 (five) days!

I know you are smart now, but you can become even smarter. I know the secret and I will share it with you, if you promise not to give up after the first or second day. I will prove to you that you can be smarter if you follow my instructions for five days.

"WHAT'S THE SECRET?" you ask.

It's so simple, you can easily do it.

Yes . . . you, you, you!

Oh, I almost forgot to tell you . . . In order to be smarter in 5 days, you MUST believe in yourself. What good is being smarter if you don't believe *you are smart already?*

What I'm offering you is a chance to be smarter than you are right now. Being smart usually takes a long time, but my method will take only 5 days!!!

First, I must be honest and tell you that you must sign the pledge on the next page to prove that you are really brave enough to succeed. After signing the pledge, fold the page and put it in an envelope. Then give it to me in exchange for the Prime-Time Smartness Challenge Materials.

DO NOT TURN THE PAGE UNTIL YOU HAVE READ THIS PAGE CAREFULLY!

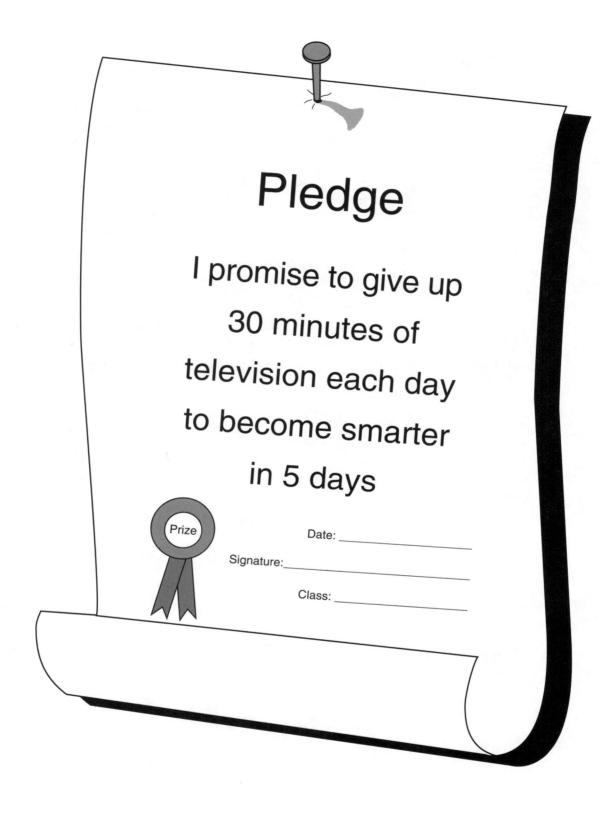

Pledge

I promise to give up
30 minutes of
television each day
to become smarter
in 5 days

Prize

Date: _____

Signature:_____

Class: _____

My Favorite Prime-Time Shows

Directions

Write the names of three of your favorite television shows on the lines below each day of the week.

Monday

1. _____
2. _____
3. _____

Tuesday

1. _____
2. _____
3. _____

Wednesday

1. _____
2. _____
3. _____

Thursday

1. _____
2. _____
3. _____

Friday

1. _____
2. _____
3. _____

Name _____

Class _____

Prime-Time Smartness Challenge Materials

Hello Again!
Did you follow the instructions? Great! Now you will begin the real test. Are you ready to follow the steps below? Good luck! See you in the winner's circle!!

Step 1

List the names of the shows (one each day) that you agree to give up to become smarter. Look at "My Favorite Prime-Time Shows" if you don't remember which ones you chose.

Step 2

Here comes the real secret. Are you ready? Turn the page to **The Star Page**. On that page there is a passage for you to read. Please look it over, then go on to Step 3.

Step 3

Now that you have seen **The Star Page**, here's what you do. . . . Each day, instead of watching one of your favorite television programs, you agree to read **The Star Page** three times, then do some other activity. You must read each word. If you skip a word, start over. Remember, read this page instead of watching one of your favorite shows.

Step 4

Keep track of your success on the "Prime-Time Smartness Challenge" page. Return it and **The Questions Page** to your teacher after the week is over.

IS GIVING UP 30 MINUTES OF TELEVISION TOO MUCH TO ASK TO GET SMARTER?

The Star Page

ECHIDNAS (E-KID-NAS)

Echidnas are egg-laying mammals. The female deposits a single egg in her pouch while lying on her back. The egg hatches about ten days later, but a young echidna stays in its mother's pouch and feeds from milk "patches" until its spines begin to develop. An echidna's spines are its protection. If threatened, the animal curls up in a ball, offering a mouthful of sharp spines to other animal attackers. On soft soil, it will use its long foreclaws to bury itself and escape heat and disturbances. The echidna has short legs, but they are very powerful. The animal can dig a hole rapidly in soft or hard ground.

Prime-Time Smartness Challenge

Put a check in the box next to each day that you succeed in following your pledge:

☐ **Day 1:** I gave up watching _____. Instead, I read The Star Page three times. For the rest of the 30 minutes I _____ _____. (Ideas: played a game, danced to music, drew, helped a family member with something he or she was doing.)

☐ **Day 2:** I gave up watching _____. I read The Star Page three times, then I _____ for the rest of the 30 minutes.

☐ **Day 3:** I'm halfway there—I know I can make it! I gave up watching _____ _____. After I read The Star Page three times, I _____.

☐ **Day 4:** I'm getting smarter—I can feel it. I gave up watching _____ _____. I read The Star Page three times, then I _____.

☐ **Day 5:** I gave up watching _____. Instead, I did my best to fill out The Questions Page. Now I am finished with the Prime-Time Smartness Challenge!

? The Questions Page ?

(Save for Day 5)

1. By now, you have learned many facts about echidnas. Please list four (or more if you can)! *(Tonight, go to someone in your home and tell him or her one interesting fact that you have learned).*

    1. _____

    2. _____

    3. _____

    4. _____

2. If someone said that an echidna would make a great pet, would you agree? (Why or why not?) Write a short paragraph explaining your answer.

    _____

    _____

    _____

    _____

    _____

Eat Well & *Keep Moving* **101**

RETA E. KING LIBRARY

CONGRATULATIONS!
YOU'RE A WINNER!

_____

Student's Name

Do you feel smarter? Did you know about echidnas before you started this assignment? Think of all you've learned!

You can give up TV for 30 minutes each day!

Keep up the good work!

Freeze My TV Summary

Freeze My TV, an extension activity to lesson 8 (Prime-Time Smartness), challenges students to keep track of and limit the amount of time they spend watching television in a designated week.

For each day of an entire seven-day week, students will log the number of hours they spend viewing television, watching videotapes, and playing video games. By keeping track of their own viewing habits, students can then see how they compare to other youth their age as well as to the *American Academy of Pediatrics'* recommended goal of watching no more than two hours of television per day.

In addition to logging television-viewing time, other contest activities include graphing, chart development, and journal writing.

Objectives

1. To have fourth- and fifth-grade students keep track of the time they spend watching television for a week, and to use this information and experience to develop graphs and write journal entries.

2. To have fourth- and fifth-grade students try to limit the time they spend viewing television to no more than two hours each day.

3. To have students think of alternative ways (especially physically active ways) they could spend their time other than watching television. Examples include playing a game, doing a puzzle, reading, talking with friends, singing and dancing to music, helping with chores, moving around, or writing songs or poems.

Materials

Materials for the *Freeze My TV* promotion are included in lesson 25.

Chain-Five

Background

Most fruits and vegetables are naturally low in fat and provide many essential nutrients and other food components important for health. These foods are excellent sources of vitamin C, vitamin B_6, carotenoids (including those that form vitamin A), folate (folic acid), and fiber. The antioxidant nutrients found in plant foods (e.g., vitamin C, carotenoids, vitamin E, and certain minerals) are currently of great interest to scientists because of their potentially beneficial role in reducing the risk of cancer and certain other chronic diseases. Scientists are also trying to determine if other substances in plant foods protect against cancer.

The GET 3-AT-SCHOOL & 5-A-DAY promotion, which encourages students to eat more fruits and vegetables, can be used as an extension to this lesson. See lesson 26 in part III, Promotions for the Classroom, for details.

The availability of fresh fruits and vegetables varies by season and region of the country. However, frozen and canned fruits and vegetables are affordable, healthful options that are available throughout the year. The goal is to eat at least five servings of fruits and vegetables a day.

Estimated Teaching Time and Related Subject Areas

Estimated teaching time: 65 minutes

Related subject areas: science, language arts, art

Objectives

1. Students will identify the benefits of consuming a variety of fruits and vegetables each day as well as other foods high in vitamins and minerals.
2. Students will explain how vitamins and minerals obtained from food in these groups contribute to a healthy body.

Materials

1. Blackboard
2. Pencil case (storage box) or school supply box containing transparent tape, chalk, erasers, ruler, pencils, pens, post-it notes
3. Pictures of fruits and vegetables
4. Transparency #1, "Fruit and Vegetable Labels"
5. Transparency #2, "Mineral Food Labels"
6. Worksheet #1, "Chain-Five: Vitamins and Minerals"
7. Worksheet #2, "Vitamins and Minerals Chart"

Procedure

1. Display the contents of storage case/box and explain to the class, "This is the case/box where I get my supplies. These are the things I need to write on the board, to mark papers, to repair papers, and to write notes to identify pages I want to find quickly. My supply box is important to me because it contains things I need. It also works for me by keeping all the things I need together so that they will be ready for use. I must constantly put new things in my storage box. Can anyone tell me why?"

   Students' possible answers:

   - When pencils are used a lot they get shorter and the erasers get smaller.
   - All the paper is used up on the "post-it" page.
   - New supplies must be put in so that they will never run out.

   Respond: "All of the things in the box have a job to do. They are useful to me and help me do the job I must do. Sometimes they work together. For example, I need my "post-it" notepad and my pen to make notes when reading pages in the teacher's guide. In my red pen there's an ink cartridge that contains the ink I need in order to correct your papers."

2. Explain: "Fruits and vegetables are like the supplies in my container because they are sources of things our bodies need. These 'things' are called nutrients (vitamins, minerals, and other nutrients), which are substances our bodies need to be healthy; and just as I need to replace my supplies when they run low, we need to replace the nutrients in our bodies because our bodies use them every day."

3. Ask the class what they think is the most popular breakfast juice. Acknowledge all answers, and ask the following question when "orange juice" is given as an answer: "What is the primary vitamin found in oranges?" (Vitamin C)

   Explain that an orange is a "citrus fruit" and ask if the students can name other fruits that belong in this group (grapefruit, limes, lemons, tangerines, tangelos).

4. Tell the students that other sources of vitamin C include broccoli, cantaloupes, peppers, tomatoes, and baked potatoes.

5. Write the word "vitamins" on the board. Have students discuss what they know about vitamins.

   Possible answers:

   - Vitamins are things your body needs to stay healthy.
   - Vitamins are listed on cans, bags, boxes of food.
   - Vitamin pills are purchased and taken by mouth.

Key Ideas

- Vitamins are important for growth and maintenance of the body.
- Vitamins do not work alone. They work with other nutrients to get a job done.
- When we eat foods containing vitamins, some are broken down, used, and excreted by the body, while others are stored by the body.
- Vitamins help to reduce the risk of certain chronic diseases, for example, certain cancers and heart disease.
- Vitamin C helps the body maintain healthy tissue, healthy skin, and healthy blood vessels.

6. Display pictures of dark green, leafy vegetables and yellow-orange colored vegetables. Explain to students: "These foods contain lots of vitamin A. This vitamin enables us to see at night and gives us healthy skin."

7. Show the "Fruit and Vegetable Labels" transparency (one label for a fruit selection and one for a vegetable selection). Ask the students to identify vitamins listed on the label of each selection.

8. Have students suggest reasons why a variety of fruits and vegetables must be eaten daily.

   Sample reasons:

   • Foods/nutrients work together to keep the body healthy.

   • There is more than one source of the same nutrient.

   • Many different substances are needed to bring about chemical reactions in the body.

   • Not all nutrients are contained in one food selection.

9. Display a photograph or a container of milk and explain, "It is important to eat a variety of fruits and vegetables so you get all the vitamins you need. It is also important to eat a variety of foods so that you get all the minerals you need. Like vitamins, minerals are substances that keep your body strong and working well. For example, milk has a lot of calcium, which is a mineral. Calcium is important for bones and teeth."

10. Write the word "minerals" on the board and list some important ones. Also explain how each is helpful to the body.

Table 9.1   Minerals

Calcium helps keep bones and teeth strong	**Zinc** helps our body get energy from the food we eat
Iron helps blood carry oxygen to all parts of the body	**Potassium** helps our nerves function and our muscles, especially the heart, work properly
Iodine helps our body get energy from the food we eat	

11. Explain to the class that we get some minerals from fruits and vegetables, but we also get minerals from other sources, such as milk (and milk products like cheese and yogurt) and lean meat. It is important to eat a balanced diet to make sure we get all the vitamins and minerals we need.

12. Show the "Mineral Food Labels" transparency to the class. Ask the students to identify minerals listed on the label of each food selection. Remember: if the % Daily Value number is 5 or less, the food is low in that nutrient.

13. Have the students form pairs or small groups. Distribute "Chain-Five" worksheet and "Vitamins and Minerals Chart." Have pairs/small groups use the chart to identify a fruit or vegetable for each vitamin in the first chain and a food source for each mineral in the second chain. Suggest that they select fruits, vegetables, and other foods that they enjoy.

14. As the groups are working, distribute strips of paper (at least five of each color per group) and paste, tape, or staplers. Once the groups have completed the worksheet,

have them write one of the vitamins (including the extra one they chose for the fifth box) on each of the strips of color #1, with the fruit or vegetable source on the back. On the strips of color #2, have them write each of the minerals, with the food source they chose on the back.

15. Have each group link their strips together into paper chains, either alternating or grouping colors. You may want to link all of the groups' chains into one to hang up in the classroom, or leave them in shorter lengths to decorate various areas of the room.

16. Explain to students that the chain is a visual reminder that it is important to eat a variety of fruits and vegetables (at least five servings each day), and other foods in order to get all of the vitamins and minerals they need for healthy bodies.

Fruit and Vegetable Labels

Plums	
Nutrition Facts	
Serving Size 2 medium	
Amount Per Serving	
Calories 80	Calories from Fat 10
	% Daily Value*
Total Fat 1g	**1%**
Saturated Fat 0g	**0%**
Cholesterol 0mg	**0%**
Sodium 0mg	**0%**
Potassium 220mg	**6%**
Total Carbohydrate 19g	**6%**
Dietary Fiber 2g	**8%**
Sugars 21g	
Protein 1g	
Vitamin A 6% • Vitamin C 20%	
Calcium 0% • Iron 0%	

*Percent Daily Values are based on a 2,000 calorie diet. Your daily values may be higher or lower depending on your calorie needs.
**Contains less than 2% of the Daily Value of these nutrients.

Sweet Potatoes	
Nutrition Facts	
Serving Size 1 medium	
Amount Per Serving	
Calories 130	Calories from Fat 0
	% Daily Value*
Total Fat 0g	**0%**
Saturated Fat 0g	**0%**
Cholesterol 0mg	**0%**
Sodium 45mg	**2%**
Potassium 350mg	**10%**
Total Carbohydrate 33g	**11%**
Dietary Fiber 4g	**16%**
Sugars 7g	
Protein 2g	
Vitamin A 440% • Vitamin C 30%	
Calcium 2% • Iron 2%	

*Percent Daily Values are based on a 2,000 calorie diet. Your daily values may be higher or lower depending on your calorie needs.
**Contains less than 2% of the Daily Value of these nutrients.

Mineral Food Labels

Skim Milk

Nutrition Facts

Serving Size 1/2 pint (236 ml)
Servings Per Container 1

Amount Per Serving

Calories 90	Calories from Fat 0

% Daily Value*

Total Fat 0g	**0%**
Saturated Fat 0g	**0%**
Cholesterol <5mg	**1%**
Sodium 130mg	**5%**
Total Carbohydrate 13g	**4%**
Dietary Fiber 0g	**0%**
Sugars 12g	
Protein 9g	

Vitamin A 10%	•	Vitamin C 2%
Calcium 30%	•	Iron 0%

*Percent Daily Values are based on a 2,000 calorie diet. Your daily values may be higher or lower depending on your calorie needs.

**Contains less than 2% of the Daily Value of these nutrients.

Chicken

Nutrition Facts

Serving Size 1 roasted drumstick
(61 g/about 2 oz.)
Servings Per Container 6

Amount Per Serving

Calories 110	Calories from Fat 50

% Daily Value*

Total Fat 6g	**9%**
Saturated Fat 1.5g	**8%**
Cholesterol 85mg	**28%**
Sodium 50mg	**2%**
Total Carbohydrate 0g	**0%**
Protein 14g	**28%**
Iron	**4%**

Not a significant source of dietary Fiber, Sugars, Vitamin A, Vitamin C, or Calcium

*Percent Daily Values are based on a 2,000 calorie diet. Your daily values may be higher or lower depending on your calorie needs.

**Contains less than 2% of the Daily Value of these nutrients.

Chain-Five: Vitamins and Minerals

Name _____ Date _____

Part A. Directions

Use the Vitamins and Minerals Chart to identify fruits and vegetables for each vitamin in the chain below. In the last box of the chain, choose any fruit or vegetable you would like and write in a vitamin it provides.

Vitamins

| Vitamin C | Vitamin A | Folate | Vitamin B2 | |

Food sources:

_____ + _____ + _____ + _____ + _____

Part B. Directions

Use the Vitamins and Minerals Chart to identify a food source for each mineral in the chain below.

Minerals

| Calcium | Iron | Potassium | Zinc | |

Food sources:

_____ + _____ + _____ + _____ + _____

Vitamins and Minerals Chart

Table 9.2   **Vitamins and Minerals Chart**

What's the Nutrient?	Where Can I Get it?
Vitamins	
Vitamin A	Carrots, sweet potatoes, greens, kale, spinach
Vitamin C	Oranges, grapefruit, tangerines, broccoli, bell peppers, tomatoes, potatoes
Vitamin D	Vitamin D fortified milk, salmon, egg yolk
Vitamin E	Seed oils, corn oil, milk
Vitamin K	Green leafy vegetables, broccoli, cabbage, turnip greens, kale, sardines
Folate	Dried beans, green leafy vegetables, kale, spinach, yeast, soybeans, wheat germ, orange juice
B vitamins: such as B1 (Thiamine) B2 (Riboflavin)	Liver, wheat (breakfast cereals), lean meat, yogurt, low-fat milk, eggs
Minerals	
Calcium	Low-fat milk, low-fat cheese, yogurt, cottage cheese, broccoli
Potassium	Bananas, oranges, apricots, avocados, potatoes, bran, peanuts, dried beans, and lean meat
Iron	Lean meat, whole-wheat bread, spinach, liver
Zinc	Lean meat, seafood, whole wheat bread, eggs, liver
Iodine	Seafood

Alphabet Fruit (and Vegetables)

Background

This lesson helps teach students the importance of eating at least five servings of fruits and vegetables a day. Leading health authorities recommend that both adults and children eat *at least* five servings of fruits and vegetables daily. Getting 5-A-Day can help reduce the risk of cancer, diabetes, heart disease, and obesity. It's especially important to get children excited early on about getting 5-A-Day so that they establish healthy eating patterns that will last a lifetime.

The GET 3-AT-SCHOOL & 5-A-DAY promotion, which encourages students to eat more fruits and vegetables, can be used as an extension to this lesson. See lesson 26 in part III, Promotions for the Classroom, for details.

Helping Your Kids Get 5-A-Day

Parents and guardians are crucial partners in this task. Photocopying and sharing with parents the handout "Helping Your Kids Get Their 5-A-Day" (page 119) will help reinforce the messages of this lesson (as well as others in the Eat Well & *Keep Moving* curriculum). Suggest that parents try one tip each week (or each day, if they seem particularly motivated).

Parental involvement is a very important component of the Eat Well & *Keep Moving* program. For more detailed information about potential parent-student activities, see "Parent and Community Involvement Guide" on the CD-ROM.

1. **Make more seem like less:** 5-A-Day sounds like a lot unless you divide them up throughout the day—e.g., one at breakfast (orange juice), one at lunch (carrot or celery sticks), one as a snack (apple or banana), and two at dinner (a salad and a baked potato). That equals five!

2. **Bring out the cook in you:** Get your child involved with the shopping *and preparation* of fruits and vegetables for your family. Ask your child to arrange a fruit plate for dessert or a vegetable tray for a party. The more your child helps in the preparation, the more likely he/she is to eat it.

3. **Dip it, dunk it:** Fruits and vegetables taste better to kids when combined with low-fat dips and dressings.

4. **Crunchy munchies:** Raw produce is the preferred choice over cooked fruits and vegetables. Serve the kids crunchy munchies—apples, pears, carrots, broccoli, celery, and cucumbers, among others.

5. **Explore the unknown:** Most children are afraid to try new fruits and vegetables. Try to offer them a wide variety of fruits and vegetables at an early age. Keep offering those fruits and vegetables to help prevent later dislikes.

6. **Set an example:** Children model what they see their parents and teachers do. If parents and teachers eat plenty of fruits and vegetables, they're more likely to as well.

7. **Gimme more:** Serve up a few different vegetables at dinner—a couple that they are familiar with and one or two that are new.

8. **Benefits:** Tell the kids how eating fruits and vegetables will make them look and feel better. Eating 5-A-Day *may* help keep cancer away!

9. **Masquerade your mango:** Turn disgust into delicious with a disguise. Smell, color, and texture are three important qualities that can turn kids on or off to fruit and vegetables.

Combine fruits and vegetables with their favorite foods. For instance, drizzle melted low-fat cheese on top of cauliflower.

This lesson will include the five parts of a safe workout and a nutrition concept (5-A-Day: fruits and vegetables). Students will be moving during the lesson, which will stress the importance of how both exercise and eating right help take care of the body! It's a team effort!

Estimated Teaching Time and Related Subject Area

Estimated teaching time: 60 minutes

Related subject area: language arts

Objectives

1. Students will learn about a variety of fruits and vegetables.
2. Students will understand and be able to describe the importance of eating at least five fruits and vegetables a day.
3. Students will demonstrate the safe workout and its five parts.

Materials

1. Handout #1, "Helping Your Kids Get Their 5-A-Day" (provided)
2. Five sets of Fruit and Vegetable cards (provided)
3. Five containers (e.g., bags, boxes) in which to put the cards

Procedure

1. Ask the students if they have eaten any fruits or vegetables today.
2. Ask the students to create a 5-A-Day menu for themselves. Ask them: "What fruit or vegetable could you have for breakfast? lunch? snack? dinner? Did you eat five today? More? Less?"
3. Discuss the reasons we need to eat 5-A-Day. For example, fruits and vegetables aid in preventing cancer and heart disease; they help the body heal wounds and burns; they prevent and fight infections; and they promote good dental health. Fruits and vegetables are also low in fat, sodium, and calories.
4. Lead students through a warm-up and stretch.

   Warm-up: the first part of the safe workout, in which slow movements get the body ready for stretching and the fitness activity.

   Stretch: the part of the safe workout in which you do exercises that improve flexibility fitness and get the body ready for the fitness activity.
5. Explain to students that they are going to participate in a fitness activity focusing on fruits and vegetables.

   Fitness activity: the part of the safe workout in which strength and endurance fitness exercises are performed.
6. Have the class form five groups.

7. Review the names of the fruits and vegetables on the cards.

8. Place the fruit and vegetable cards in a "bag" in front of each group.

9. Set aside a place on the floor on the opposite side of the classroom where each group can put their fruit and vegetable cards in alphabetical order.

10. The students will be moving nonstop (either walking or jogging in place) behind the card container. On the signal by the teacher, the first person will get a card and go to the opposite side of the room, put the card down in the designated space, go back to the group and give a "high five" to the next student. The next student in line will then pick up a card, place it on the floor in alphabetical order, and go back to the group.

11. This will continue until all fruit and vegetable cards are in alphabetical order on the floor.

12. This can be done more than once depending on time.

13. Lead students in a cool-down and cool-down stretch.

    Cool-down: the part of the safe workout in which your body slows down and recovers from the fitness activity.

    Cool-down stretch: the last part of the safe workout in which you do exercises that improve flexibility fitness.

14. Guide students through the "Stay Healthy Corner":

    a. Have each group check to make sure the cards are in alphabetic order. Then have them pick five cards and discuss how these five could fit into their daily meals and snacks.

    b. Discuss some tips on how students can get five fruits and vegetables a day (see "Helping Your Kids Get Their 5-A-Day" for ideas, page 119) and ask them to offer their own experiences. For example, they might say, "My mom gives me money to pick out any fruits and vegetables I want;" "I like baked potatoes and sour cream;" "I like having orange juice for breakfast;" "Sometimes grown-ups don't set the right example—they don't eat fruits and vegetables."

    c. Encourage the students to give advice as to how the class can eat more fruits and vegetables each day.

Have students take their handout "Helping Your Kids Get Their 5-A-Day" home and post it on the refrigerator. Suggest that they work with their parents to try one tip every week (maybe even every day).

Helping Your Kids Get Their 5-A-Day

1. **Make more seem like less:** 5-A-Day sounds like a lot unless you divide them up throughout the day—e.g., one at breakfast (orange juice), one at lunch (carrot or celery sticks), one as a snack (apple or banana), and two at dinner (a salad and a baked potato). That equals five!

2. **Bring out the cook in you:** Get your child involved with the shopping *and preparation* of fruits and vegetables for your family. Ask your child to arrange a fruit plate for dessert or a vegetable tray for a party. The more your child helps in the preparation, the more likely he/she is to eat it.

3. **Dip it, dunk it:** Fruits and vegetables taste better to kids when combined with low-fat dips and dressings.

4. **Crunchy munchies:** Raw produce is the preferred choice over cooked fruits and vegetables. Serve the kids crunchy munchies—apples, pears, carrots, broccoli, celery, and cucumbers, among others.

5. **Explore the unknown:** Most children are afraid to try new fruits and vegetables. Try to offer them a wide variety of fruits and vegetables at an early age. Keep offering those fruits and vegetables to help prevent later dislikes.

6. **Set an example:** Children model what they see their parents and teachers do. If parents and teachers eat plenty of fruits and vegetables, they're more likely to as well.

7. **Gimme more:** Serve up a few different vegetables at dinner—a couple that they are familiar with and one or two that are new.

8. **Benefits:** Tell the kids how eating fruits and vegetables will make them look and feel better. Eating 5-A-Day *may* help keep cancer away!

9. **Masquerade your mango:** Turn disgust into delicious with a disguise. Smell, color, and texture are three important qualities that can turn kids on or off to fruit and vegetables.

   Combine fruits and vegetables with their favorite foods. For instance, drizzle melted low-fat cheese on top of cauliflower.

apples	apricots
artichokes	avocados
bananas	beets
berries	bok choy
broccoli	brussels sprouts

cabbage	carrots
cauliflower	celery
cherries	coconuts
collards	corn
cucumbers	dates

eggplant	figs
grapes	grapefruit
green beans	green peppers
kale	kelp
kiwi	kumquats

lemons	lettuce
limes	mangoes
melons	mushrooms
nectarines	okra
onions	oranges

papayas	parsnips
peaches	pears
peas	peppers
persimmons	pineapples
plums	prunes

pumpkins	radishes
raisins	romaine lettuce
spinach	squash
sweet potatoes	Swiss chard
tangerines	tomatoes

turnips	zucchini

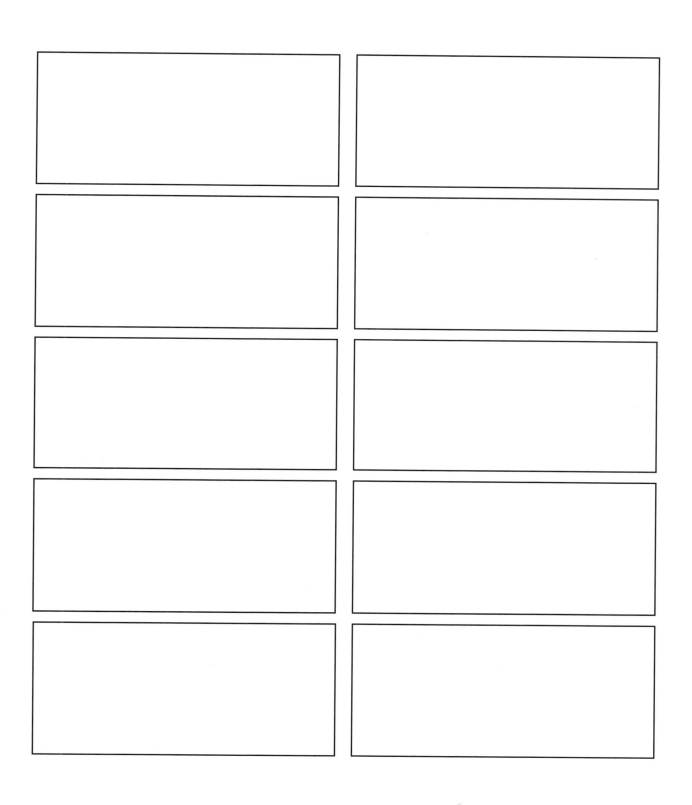

Brilliant Breakfast*

Background**

Breakfast is the most important meal of the day. Eating breakfast gives the body the energy it needs to start the day and perform the morning's important tasks, from thinking to doing the dishes to working out. Generally, adults who regularly eat breakfast learned this lifelong good habit when they were children.

Studies show that children who eat breakfast are better prepared for the school day. They perform better in school, are tardy less often, and miss fewer days of school. Students who eat breakfast have also demonstrated that their ability to concentrate is better, their reaction times are faster, their energy levels are higher, and their scores on tests are better.

To help make breakfast a lifelong habit, students (and adults) should be encouraged to start their day by eating breakfast. Any good, nutritious food can be eaten for breakfast. If people don't happen to like typical breakfast foods, such as cereal or toast, they can eat leftovers from dinner, like pizza or a sandwich. The most important thing is to eat a nutritious meal in the morning.

Ideally, breakfast should contain a substantial amount of carbohydrates (from foods like whole grain cereal, toast, fruit, and 100% fruit juice—but not from foods made with refined or processed sugars, like soda and candy) and some protein (preferably from nuts or low-fat dairy like 1% milk and low-fat yogurt). This means eating from the bottom three layers of the Food Guide Pyramid—the grain group, fruits and vegetables groups, and low-fat dairy and protein groups.

The carbohydrates in a nutritious breakfast give the body energy, and the protein helps stave off a midmorning drop in blood sugar level that can make children lethargic before lunchtime. Blood sugar levels indicate how much fuel (in the form of glucose) is immediately available to the body. When blood sugar levels drop, children (and adults) may feel drowsy, feel less energetic, and have trouble concentrating. Breakfast can help keep blood sugar levels up throughout the morning until lunchtime.

Foods such as doughnuts, colas, candy bars, and desserts contain a lot of simple sugars and are not the best choices for breakfast because they can cause blood sugar levels to drop faster than foods containing complex carbohydrates and protein.

* Adapted, by permission, from the Texas Education Agency. From the Texas Education Agency Nutrition Education Curriculum Guide, Grades 5-8.
** Partial source of background material: Maryland Food Committee.

Estimated Teaching Time and Related Subject Areas

Estimated teaching time: 60 minutes

Related subject areas: math, science

Objectives

1. Students will able to describe the importance of a healthful breakfast.
2. Students will identify the effects of eating a nutritious breakfast and a less-than-nutritious breakfast.
3. Students will create breakfasts to fit different lifestyles and needs.

Materials

1. Worksheet #1, "The Breakfast Club"
2. Transparency #1, "Avoid Midmorning Slump"
3. Solutions to worksheet #1

Procedure

1. Ask students to raise their hands if they like to eat breakfast.
2. Ask students if they know what the word "breakfast" means. Tell students that breakfast means "breaking the fast" and that a "fast" is when the body has gone for a long period without food—such as overnight.
3. Tell students that during a fast, the amount of sugar in the blood is reduced (the sugar eventually is transported to muscles and organs to create energy for work). When this happens, your body isn't getting all the energy it needs to work really efficiently—whether you're playing or thinking.
4. Tell students that when they eat breakfast, they are breaking the overnight fast and giving the body what it needs to work until lunchtime. On the other hand, if they skip breakfast in the morning, they may
   - be less alert;
   - be less energetic;
   - be less efficient at completing tasks;
   - experience headaches, stomach cramps, and irritability; or
   - show reduced achievement.
5. Ask students what they like to eat for breakfast. Write responses on the board. Tell students that they should all try to eat breakfast every morning, and that eating any type of nutritious food in the morning is better than eating nothing. Some foods, though, are better than others for breakfast.
6. Have students categorize the breakfast foods written on the board into the different groups of the Food Guide Pyramid.

If appropriate, remind students that *breakfast is available to them before school in the cafeteria.*

7. Tell students that the ideal breakfast should contain a lot of carbohydrates (from foods like whole grain cereal and toast, fruit, and 100% fruit juice—but not from foods made with refined or processed sugars, like soda and candy) and some protein (usually from foods likes peanut butter and low-fat milk and yogurt). The carbohydrates give the body energy, and the protein helps stave off a midmorning drop in the level of sugar in the blood (blood sugar), which can make them feel hungry, drowsy, and sluggish before lunchtime.
8. Also tell students that foods high in simple sugars (such as doughnuts, colas, candy bars, and desserts) are not ideal for breakfast because they can cause blood sugar levels to drop below fasting levels within a few hours. These types of foods also tend to contain very few other nutrients, like vitamins and minerals.
9. Distribute and review "The Breakfast Club" worksheet with the students. After students have completed the worksheet, use the "Avoid Midmorning Slump"

transparency to review their answers and show students what happens to blood sugar levels with each breakfast.

Discussion Points for Transparency:

- Breakfast #1 (the skipped breakfast) did not provide any food, so energy must come from body storage. Blood sugar levels remain at or below fasting levels.
- Breakfast #2 provides enough protein to help Tisha be alert and discourage midmorning hunger pangs and provides enough complex carbohydrates for sustained energy.
- Breakfast #3 contains too much refined sugar and not enough protein to keep blood sugar levels up until lunch. The result is a midmorning slump.

10. With the class, write several nutritious breakfast menus that address the specific situation of the people listed below.

Breakfasts for those who wake up late:

- Breakfast shakes with low-fat milk
- Milk and fruit
- Yogurt
- Leftover supper entrees
- Orange juice

Breakfasts for those who do not like typical breakfast foods:

- Wheat crackers with cheese, or peanut butter crackers
- English muffin pizzas
- Breakfast burritos
- Bacon, lettuce, and tomato sandwich

Breakfasts for Chinese children:

- Rice
- Soup
- Vegetables
- Beans (soybeans)
- Fish (baked/boiled)

Breakfasts for Brazilian children:

- Chocolate milk
- Sweet rolls with butter
- Fresh fruit (bananas, guava, mango, grapes)

Breakfasts for children from Ghana:

- Soup/stew
- Rice
- Plantains

11. Instruct students to create their own nutritious, energizing breakfasts based on their own lifestyles, traditions, and food preferences. Ask some of them to share their breakfast menus with the class.

The Breakfast Club

Name_____ Date_____

Breakfast

Jeremy's Breakfast

Jeremy was late for school, so he left without eating breakfast. By midmorning (around 10:00 A.M.), he was fidgety and had trouble concentrating. His stomach was grumbling before lunchtime, and he had trouble completing his morning math quiz.

Tisha's Breakfast

Tisha was also running late for school, but when she got there, she went to the cafeteria and ate the school breakfast of 100% juice, pancakes, and 1% milk. She felt great all morning and did very well on her math quiz.

Omar's Breakfast

Omar grabbed two doughnuts and a glass of Kool-Aid as he ran out the door for school. He was full of energy and enthusiasm for a while, then his mind started to wander, and, like Jeremy, he had trouble finishing the math quiz.

Why did Jeremy, Tisha, and Omar feel the way they did by lunchtime?

1._____

_____

_____

2._____

_____

_____

3._____

_____

_____

Avoid Midmorning Slump

A good breakfast should have a lot of complex carbohydrates (approximately 40 grams) and some protein (12-18 grams). This combination helps the body avoid a midmorning slump in energy.

You can see how many grams of protein or carbohydrates there are in a food by looking at its food label.

When blood sugar drops below the fasting level, a person may have a harder time concentrating on school work, may feel light-headed, and may be less alert.

Jeremy's breakfast:

Breakfast #1
Skips morning meal
Energy must come from body
storage

Carbohydrate: 0 grams
Protein: 0 grams

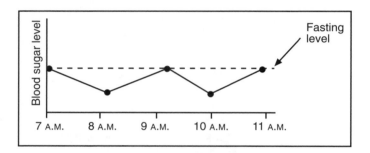

Tisha's breakfast:

Breakfast #2
Optimal morning meal example
2 pancakes
8 oz 1% milk
1/2 cup 100% orange juice

Carbohydrate: 45 grams
Protein: 7 grams

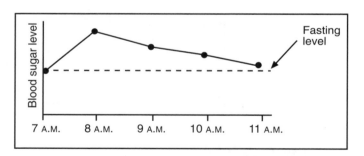

Omar's breakfast:

Breakfast #3
High-carbohydrate morning meal example
2 doughnuts
1/2 cup Kool-Aid

Carbohydrate: 37 grams
Protein: 2 grams

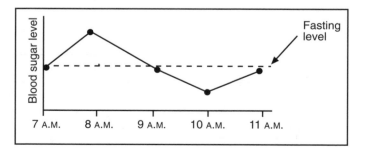

Solutions

Worksheet 1   The Breakfast Club

Breakfast

Jeremy's Breakfast

Jeremy was late for school, so he left without eating breakfast. By midmorning (around 10:00 A.M.), he was fidgety and had trouble concentrating. His stomach was grumbling before lunchtime, and he had trouble completing his morning math quiz.

Tisha's Breakfast

Tisha was also running late for school, but when she got there, she went to the cafeteria and ate the school breakfast of 100% juice, pancakes, and 1% milk. She felt great all morning and did very well on her math quiz.

Omar's Breakfast

Omar grabbed two doughnuts and a glass of Kool-Aid as he ran out the door for school. He was full of energy and enthusiasm for a while, then his mind started to wander, and, like Jeremy, he had trouble finishing the math quiz.

Why did Jeremy, Tisha, and Omar feel the way they did by lunchtime?

1. Jeremy did not eat anything in the morning. He did not break his overnight fast so his energy needed to come from body storage. This kept his blood sugar levels low, making him hungry, lethargic, and distracted.

2. Tisha ate an excellent breakfast with a lot of grains (pancakes), some 100% fruit juice, and some protein (from the 1% milk.) This breakfast kept her blood sugar up at normal levels throughout the morning, keeping her alert and energized until lunch time.

3. It was good that Omar ate a breakfast. However, his breakfast was not ideal. He ate foods that were too high in sugar. With so much sugar (and no milk to provide some protein), Omar felt tired and restless around midmorning because his blood sugar dropped.

Fitness Walking

Background

Walking is one of the healthiest, safest, and easiest ways to begin a fitness program and can be a big step toward improving your health. Fitness or aerobic walking uses all of the major muscle groups in the upper and lower body in a nonimpacting, dynamic, rhythmic action, which is what an ideal exercise should do.

Walking is also free! There are no machines or membership fees, no fancy packaging or expensive clothes. Walking requires only that you "race" yourself and do your "personal best." What's important is feeling good about yourself and setting your own standards and goals.

Walking can be done with friends or family. It can also be done as an adventure with a school class. An active lifestyle can make you feel better, give you more energy, and enhance your health. We want you and your class to get hooked on walking. It's fun, and it's good for you!

Overview

This lesson introduces students to the benefits and fun of walking for fitness. The lesson also serves as a kickoff for an ongoing class-walking club that can be integrated into geography activities throughout the year.

Estimated Teaching Time and Related Subject Areas

Estimated teaching time: 1 hour

Related subject areas: science, social studies, math, physical education

Objectives

1. Students will learn about the importance of regular exercise and establish an ongoing class-walking club.
2. Students will be exposed to the benefits of walking with family, friends, and classmates.
3. Students will learn walking techniques and learn about the health benefits of raising one's heart rate through regular aerobic activity.
4. Students will learn about a particular geographic region of the world.

Materials

1. Comfortable shoes (students and teacher)
2. Worksheet #1, "Teacher Classroom Walking Log"
3. Worksheet #2, "Student Classroom Walking Log" (duplicate for students)
4. Worksheet #3, "Student Home Walking Log" (duplicate for students)
5. Map(s)
6. Map pins/thumb tacks

Planning a Walking Club

In addition to introducing students to how important and fun walking can be, this lesson also focuses on the organization of a class-walking club.

When planning a walking club, first consider where and when your students can walk. The walks can take place before, during, or after school, and can be done in the hallways, gym, playgrounds, or around the neighborhood—whenever and wherever such a program works best for your school.

An effective way to introduce a walking club into your school would be to integrate it with your curriculum. One option is to integrate the club with your social studies curriculum, for example, with lessons on the state in which you live, the entire United States, or other countries around the world. If there is an area of the world your students would like to learn about, use the walking club to help you accomplish this. As a class or individually, design the itinerary of a "fitness walk" across the region you have chosen to cover. Students could walk across America together, walk across a region of the U.S., or walk around the world. The design is completely open.

Give your program a name, such as "Walk Across America" or "Walk Across the World," or let the students choose a name.

Using maps of the area(s) you choose, tie in the students' walking progress with movement on the map. Each time the class walks a certain period of time, equate that with a particular distance on the map (for example, five minutes walked could equal 50 miles). Each student can have a map, or all of the students can plot their travels on one map. The amount of time the class walks and the distance traveled will depend on the part of the world or country on which you chose to focus. For example, if you decide on a large area of the world, such as Africa, then five minutes might equal 200 miles traveled. If you chose the state of Maryland, five minutes might equal 50 miles.

Keep track of your class walks on the logs provided. There is a log for each class, as well as for each student. The class log can be made larger and displayed in the classroom for all to see. A map of the area/region/country that they will be traveling across should be displayed along with the log. Displaying the map and log will motivate the class and keep everyone more involved.

Encourage students to take on the walking program as an after-school, family-and-friend adventure. Have the students keep a log of the dates and times of their after-school walks (see "Student Home Walking Log" sheet). They can plot their travels on the maps with pins or thumb tacks. Get the whole school involved in walking—principals, office staff, custodians, and other teachers and students can become involved. The more the students see others participating, the more they will want to become involved.

Procedure

1. Fitness Walking

Explain to students that "fitness walking" is walking at a pace (speed) that makes the heart, lungs, and blood vessels work harder than usual. This type of aerobic workout makes the heart muscle pump harder because the body's other muscles—leg and arm muscles—are working harder and need more blood to keep them going.

Blood gives muscles energy to work. When muscles work hard, such as when you're doing fitness walking, they need more energy. During exercise, the heart works harder to pump blood to these muscles. When the heart works hard, it gets stronger.

Explain to students that they can check their pulse rate before they begin exercising and again during their fitness workout in order to see firsthand how the heart muscle works harder. (See details on how to do this in the section "Finding a Pulse".)

2. Benefits of Fitness Walking

Ask students to list the benefits of fitness walking. These can include the following:

   a. Walking is an excellent and safe way to achieve aerobic conditioning. Aerobic conditioning means taking care of the heart, lungs, and blood vessels. Walking lets you do this with less wear and tear on the body compared to many other types of conditioning.
   b. Walking, like other aerobic exercises, can give you more energy and reduce fatigue.
   c. Walking can help relieve stress.
   d. Walking can improve mood and mental function.
   e. Walking can help in weight control.
   f. Walking can help slow down the progression of osteoporosis (bone loss), which can occur when one ages.
   g. Walking can be performed with friends and family.

3. How to Fitness Walk

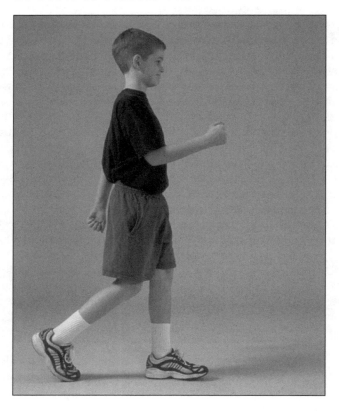

Figure 12.1 Fitness walking.

   a. Make sure students wear sneakers or comfortable shoes.
   b. Review with students the following:
      1. **Arm swing:** Try to keep the arms swinging at a pace faster than they swing when walking normally. The faster the arms swing, the faster the legs will move. Bend the arms 90 degrees at the elbow. Concentrate on moving the arms faster and swinging them from the shoulder. Remember, when you shorten your arms (bending them at the elbow 90 degrees), you can swing them faster and your legs will move faster. Keep your shoulders relaxed. Beginners tend to tense up the upper body around the shoulders. RELAX!

2. **Hands:** Form a loose fist. Do not clench your fist and put tension in the arm muscles.

3. **Foot placement and toe-off:** The power of the step comes from the toe-off action of the foot. With each step, land the foot on the heel, then roll forward to the toe and push off.

   c. Tell the students that the above information should help them to enjoy their walking more. They should do what feels comfortable for them. DO IT RIGHT, but make it FUN!

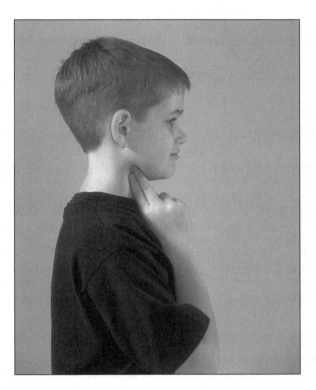

Figure 12.2 Finding a pulse.

4. The Fitness Walk

Component 1: Finding a Pulse

On the first day (or however often you would like), remind students that their pulse rate will increase when they exercise and teach them how to find their pulse. Explain the following:

   During an aerobic workout, you want your heart, lungs, and blood vessels to work harder than they are used to. Your pulse can help you know what is going on inside your body. On the side of your neck just below the jaw bone is a major blood vessel bringing blood to the brain. Put your index finger and middle finger together and place them gently on that blood vessel on the side of your neck to feel the pulse. During exercise, the pulse is usually very easy to find. (To see the change in the pulse rate from the warm-up to the fitness activity to the cool-down, it would be helpful for the students to try to feel their pulse before, during, and after aerobic walking.)

   The heart is a muscle that has a huge job to do. It must always be working, every second, minute, hour, day, week, month, and year of your lives. Once you understand that this heart muscle of yours has such a *huge* job to do, then hopefully you will want to take care of it so it can do its job.

   Walking is one way to keep the heart muscle healthy. Likewise, eating right and being active are both a big part of helping the heart stay healthy. If the heart is working harder than it's used to (feel the pulse) during the fitness activity, then with time the heart will get stronger and stay healthy. The more you include exercise and eating right in your daily lives, the better the body can work and feel!

Component 2: The Safe Workout

Following the steps of the safe workout will help you to prevent injuries. The five steps are:

Step 1: The warm-up. Start each fitness walk with a slow walk to get the body ready. Emphasize to students the importance of warming-up and stretching before doing any type of physical activity. During the warm-up, talk about the "adventure" for the day. Review the important facts about the warm-up. (Refer to lesson 3, "The Safe Workout: An Introduction.")

Step 2: The stretch. After the warm-up, stretch out and work on flexibility fitness. Review the importance of stretching and the key parts of safe stretching.

Step 3: Fitness activity. Introduce the fitness-walking activity you have chosen for your class, such as walking the first leg of a trip across the U.S. Have the class set a goal for that particular day. For example, the goal for the first day may be for the class to walk for five minutes without stopping. As students get used to the program, the class can set goals to walk longer and more frequently. Remember, the more days students walk, the greater the opportunity they have to learn and the more fit they will become.

Take the students on their fitness walk. During the walk, lead a discussion among students about the geographic region they are "walking through" on their program. Other topics to discuss may include nutrition and physical activity issues.

Step 4: Cool-down. After their fitness walk, have students walk more slowly to let their bodies recover. Review the benefits of the cool-down.

Step 5: Cool-down stretch. After the cool-down, have students stretch out again to prevent soreness, to improve flexibility, and to decrease their chances of injury. While they are stretching, review the benefits of the cool-down stretch and the proper way to cool down.

Step 6: The stay healthy corner. After the first walk, gather the class together and review the benefits of walking. Stress the importance of walking and the enjoyment they will get from it. Introduce and fill out together the classroom walking logs—worksheet #1, "Teacher Classroom Walking Log" and worksheet #2, "Student Classroom Walking Log."

Introduce and distribute worksheet #3, "Student Home Walking Log," to students. Review with them the four parts of the log sheet—(1) Date, (2) Time, (3) Miles, (4) Where—and how to complete it.

You and your students can decide how to use worksheet #3, "Student Home Walking Log." For example, students can keep track of their after-school walking program completely on their own, including tracking their progress on separate maps. Or students can integrate their after-school walking experience with their in-school tracking system.

However you approach it, the ultimate goal is to encourage and motivate students to exercise at home with family and/or friends.

Teacher Classroom Walking Log

Name _____ Class _____

Our fitness walk will take us across _____

_____

Table 12.1   Teacher Classroom Walking Log

Date	Time	Miles	Where

Date: Date of the fitness walk

Time: Number of minutes walked

Miles: Number of miles walked (depends on how many minutes your class decided equals one mile)

Where: Town, city, state, or country traveled through today

Student Classroom Walking Log

Name _____ Class _____

Our fitness walk will take us across _____

_____

Table 12.2   Student Classroom Walking Log

Date	Time	Miles	Where

Date: Date of the fitness walk

Time: Number of minutes walked

Miles: Number of miles walked (depends on how many minutes your class decided equals one mile)

Where: Town, city, state, or country traveled through today

Student Home Walking Log

Name _____ Class _____

My fitness walk will take me across _____

_____

Table 12.3   **Student Home Walking Log**

Date	Time	Miles	Where

Date: Date of the fitness walk

Time: Number of minutes walked

Miles: Number of miles walked (depends on how many minutes your class decided equals one mile)

Where: Town, city, state, or country traveled through today

Classroom Lessons for Fifth Graders

Part II includes the fifth-grade classroom lessons. Using the same multidisciplinary approach as part I, these lessons expand upon the key ideas presented in the fourth-grade lessons—emphasizing skill-building and putting knowledge into practice. With activities such as choosing healthy snacks, monitoring food choices, and limiting television time, the fifth-grade lessons provide ample opportunities for students to begin living by the themes of Eat Well & *Keep Moving*. As with the fourth-grade lessons, the key messages of the fifth-grade lessons can be bolstered by the many supporting activities of Eat Well & *Keep Moving* described in parts III-VII and the CD-ROM.

Focusing on the same broad messages of the fourth-grade lessons, these fifth-grade lessons focus on teaching students to

- eat at least five servings of fruits and vegetables a day,
- eat less fat (especially saturated and *trans* fats),
- eat a nutritious breakfast every morning,
- be more physically active, and
- be less physically inactive (specifically, reducing time spent viewing television).

Healthy Living
and the Pyramid

Background

Healthy Living

Healthy living involves making lifestyle choices that maximize our physical and mental well-being. Healthy living encompasses more than just eating a balanced diet. It also involves getting the exercise and rest our bodies need, staying away from harmful substances (such as tobacco and drugs), and engaging in activities that we enjoy and that enhance our mental well-being.

It is important to recognize that our physical health and our mental health are interrelated. For example, eating a balanced diet and exercising can not only help maintain a healthy weight, it can boost mental health by increasing energy levels and improving our ability to cope with stress. Spending time with friends can help provide support for the many challenges in life, as well as provide companions for physical activity. The key to healthy living is a balance of all aspects of life—physical, intellectual, social, and emotional.

Again, eating a balanced diet is an important component of a healthy lifestyle. Eating the right foods (plenty of fruits, vegetables, and whole grains without excess saturated and *trans* fats) provides us with the energy and nutrients our bodies need to stay healthy and helps us fight and prevent some infections and diseases. In addition, what we eat not only affects how our bodies perform and feel today, it also affects our health 10, 20, and even 30 years from now and beyond.

Healthy living means being aware of and making an effort to enhance those aspects of our lives that can keep us healthy, make us feel good, and help us lead active, full lives.

The Food Guide Pyramid

Over the years, experts have worked to form guidelines to help Americans eat better, to keep us healthier, and to enhance quality of life. The Food Guide Pyramid—a concept developed by the United States Department of Agriculture (USDA)—represents years of research on what a healthful diet should consist of for Americans over two years of age.

This research focused on what foods Americans eat now, what nutrients are in the foods we eat, and how these patterns need to change to better prevent disease and promote good health. The Food Guide Pyramid emphasizes moderation, variety, and balance. The pyramid will help you choose what and how much to eat from each food group to get the nutrients you need without getting too many calories, or too much saturated and *trans* fats, refined sugar, sodium, or alcohol.

There are six categories in the pyramid, and the size of each category corresponds to the amount of food from that group that you need to eat each day. The groups at the bottom of the pyramid take up more space, which means that you need more of these foods and less of the foods closer to the top. The food group at the tip of the pyramid is for food items that primarily consist of fat and sugar, demonstrating that it is healthy to eat these only in small amounts. For instance, a diet low in saturated and *trans* fats may help your body avoid heart disease and some types of cancer.

More than half (55%) of our daily food choices should come from the grain (especially whole grain, e.g., bread, rice, pasta), vegetable, and fruit food groups of the Food Guide Pyramid. These three food groups make up the base of a healthful, balanced diet. We all need to choose more of our foods from these three bottom groups because they provide the majority of the vitamins, minerals, and complex carbohydrates (starch and dietary fiber) needed to provide energy and to maintain good health.

Carbohydrates and Other Major Food Components

The foods that we eat contain many kinds of nutrients. Nutrients are the chemical substances in food that are used by the body to maintain health. Macronutrients

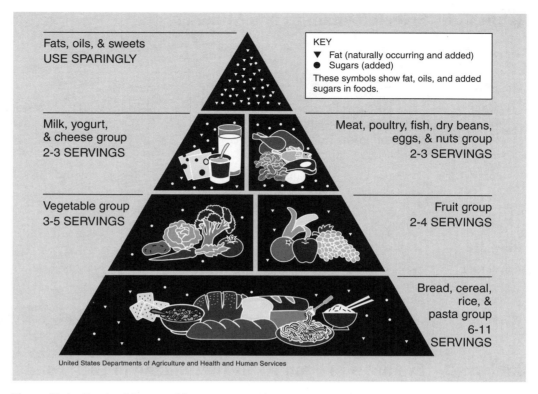

Figure 13.1 Food guide pyramid.

(carbohydrates, fats, and proteins) are the major food components. Micronutrients (vitamins and minerals) are the nutrients that we need in very small amounts and that are present in many foods. Both groups of nutrients are important for a healthy body.

All foods are made up of one, two, or all three of the macronutrients. **Protein** provides the body with the building blocks for making and repairing tissue (like muscle and skin). **Fat** helps keep the body warm, helps protect the internal organs (like the heart and liver), and helps the body transport certain vitamins. And **carbohydrates** (starches and sugars) provide the body with energy. Protein and fat can also provide energy, but carbohydrates are the quickest source of energy and the only nutrient that can be readily used for energy in every single cell in the body. Carbohydrates should be the largest part of each day's total food intake in a healthy diet.

Carbohydrates are found in many foods. The grain, fruit, and vegetable groups contain the greatest amount of carbohydrates. Whole grains, which are not refined, are preferable since they are good sources of vitamins, minerals, and fiber besides carbohydrates. The vitamins, minerals, and fiber are lost during the milling process. Other good sources include milk, yogurt, and dried beans (legumes). Sweet foods (such as soda, cookies, and candy) that contain sugar also provide carbohydrates; unfortunately, these foods usually contain very little of the micronutrients (vitamins and minerals) and can be high in saturated and *trans* fats. These foods should be eaten only in small amounts or once in a while.

Vitamins and Minerals

Vitamins and minerals are nutrients (micronutrients, specifically) needed to keep the body healthy. There are many vitamins and minerals in the foods that we eat. The following table lists some of the vitamins and minerals that are commonly low in the typical American diet. These are some of the nutrients we should be sure to get every day.

Table 13.1   Selected Vitamins and Minerals

Nutrient	Source	Role
Vitamins		
Vitamin A	dark green, yellow, and orange vegetables and fruits (such as kale, spinach, broccoli, romaine lettuce, carrots, cantaloupe, apricots), liver	Helps with night vision, bone growth, and tissue maintenance
Vitamin C	oranges, grapefruit, tangerines, cantaloupe, mangoes, papaya, strawberries, broccoli, tomatoes, bell peppers, potatoes	Keeps skin and tissue healthy
Minerals		
Calcium	low-fat milk, low-fat cheese, yogurt, cottage cheese, kale, broccoli, greens, tofu (bean curd)	Helps keep bones and teeth strong.
Iron	meat, eggs, vegetables, fortified cereals, beans	Helps carry oxygen to the cells of the body

Table 13.2   Examples of Food Items That Belong in Each Food Group

Grains	bread (corn bread, muffins, rolls, whole wheat bread, biscuits, pitas, pancakes, pretzels), cereal, oatmeal, rice, and pasta (macaroni, spaghetti)
Vegetables	collard greens, mustard greens, spinach, kale, corn, turnips, lima beans, string beans, cabbage, white potatoes, sweet potatoes, broccoli, carrots, okra, squash
Fruit	peaches, nectarines, cantaloupe, watermelon, grapefruit, raisins, apples, oranges, bananas, strawberries, pears, tangerines, grapes, pineapple
Meat, Poultry, Fish, Dry Beans, Eggs, & Nuts	peanut butter, kidney beans, navy beans, lentils, black-eyed peas, peanuts, lean meat, chicken, turkey, fish, eggs, tofu
Dairy	nonfat milk, 1% milk, 2% milk, cottage cheese, cheddar cheese, low-fat cheese, frozen yogurt

Estimated Teaching Time and Related Subject Area

Estimated Teaching Time: 1 hour, 45 minutes

Related Subject Area: science

Objectives

1. To reinforce the concept of wellness, a balanced lifestyle, and the role of carbohydrates in the diet.
2. To create a further understanding of the food groups in the Food Guide Pyramid and its recommendations.
3. To introduce the role of vitamin C and calcium in the diet.

Materials

1. Worksheet #1, "Origami Pyramid"
2. Worksheet #2, "Help! You're the Doctor"
3. Worksheet #3, "Pyramid Planning"
4. Food picture cards (often available through your state's Dairy Council) *or* pictures of food cut out from magazines (be sure to include vegetables, fruit, breads, cereals, and dairy products, which are high in carbohydrates)
5. Solutions to worksheet #2
6. Solutions to worksheet #3
7. Teacher Resource Page #1—Carbohydrate Foods
8. Teacher Resource Page #2—Low-Carbohydrate Foods

Procedure

1. Provide each student with the origami pyramid (worksheet #1) outline and have students assemble the pyramid. Discuss the six food categories and the reasons to select more foods from the base of the pyramid than from the top. On the inside of the pyramid, students can list two or three foods that belong to the base of the pyramid (grains, fruits, vegetables).
2. Explain the important roles a balanced diet and balanced lifestyle play in keeping individuals healthy.
3. Explain and discuss the role of carbohydrates, vitamin C, and calcium in the diet (see background information).
4. From the food picture cards (or foods cut out of magazines), select several foods that contain carbohydrates, vitamin C, and calcium (see background information for examples of such foods).
5. Place the cards on the board and select students to identify a food and explain the benefits of selecting that particular food to eat. Select a student to explain the function of the nutrient.
6. Distribute worksheet #2, "Help! You're the Doctor." Have students read the three cases about people who are having health concerns and answer the questions in the spaces provided on the worksheet.
7. Explain to students that "healthy living" involves ensuring that their lifestyle is balanced and varied, that it is important to eat a balanced and varied diet and to engage in a variety of activities in all aspects of their lives—social, intellectual, physical, and emotional. For example, this would include activities such as spending time with friends, reading, talking with family members, walking, dancing, running, playing sports, and even having quiet time.
8. Distribute worksheet #3, "Pyramid Planning." Review the Food Guide Pyramid concept and categories with students. Reiterate that it is important to eat more foods from the base and middle of the pyramid and fewer foods from the top of the pyramid.
9. Have students complete worksheet #3 as instructed.

Origami Pyramid

Directions

1. Using scissors, cut out the entire origami figure by cutting along the outside lines. Be sure to cut around the two round tabs at the top.

2. Fold the paper so that it forms the shape of a pyramid and tape the round tabs on the inside of the pyramid to hold it together.

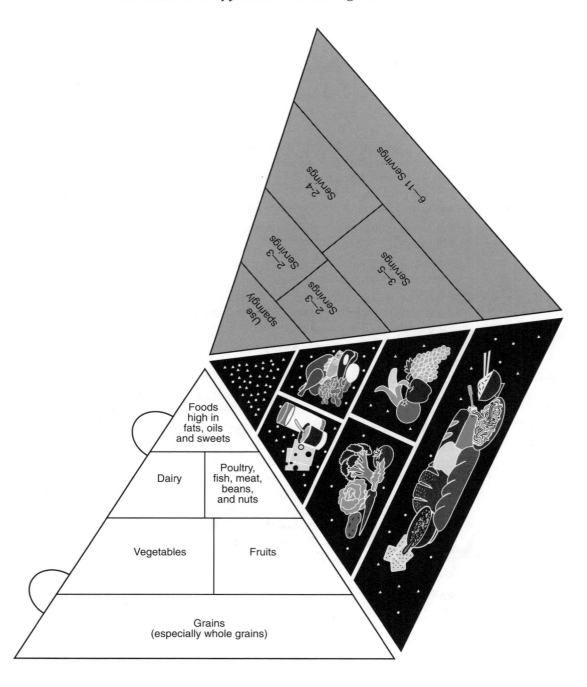

Help! You're the Doctor

Directions

Read the following paragraphs and complete the exercises.

1. Members of the Jones family have been told by a doctor that they should eat more foods that contain a lot of vitamins and minerals. The family eats a lot of foods from the grain, dairy, and protein food groups, but they obviously need a greater variety of foods in their daily diet.

   List some foods that would help the Jones family improve their diet. List five foods that contain a lot of vitamins and minerals.

   _____
   _____
   _____
   _____
   _____

2. James, a fifth-grade student, eats toast for breakfast and a meat sandwich for lunch. He eats an apple or orange each day, and always has some vegetables for his evening meal along with meat, chicken, or fish. He goes to the park or beach with his family on weekends, but during the week his only exercise is walking 150 yards from his home to his school.

   Which food group(s) is missing from James's diet? Why is this food group important? What else could James do to improve his health?

   _____
   _____
   _____
   _____
   _____

3. Maria plays basketball for two hours each afternoon at the school gym. Recently she noticed that she has no energy after the first hour, which is something that never used to happen. She has been watching a lot of television and reading books late at night, and wakes up at 6 A.M. each morning to go to school.

   List two reasons Maria may not have enough energy. How can she improve her energy level?

   _____
   _____
   _____
   _____
   _____

   Name the food groups that give us energy for action sports.

   _____
   _____
   _____

Worksheet 3

Pyramid Planning

Directions

1. Fill in the Food Guide Pyramid below with the suggested amount of servings for each group.

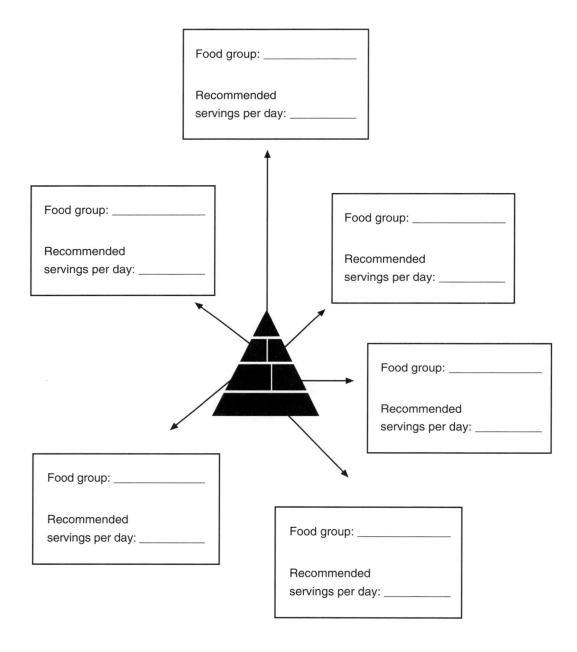

Food group: _____

Recommended
servings per day: _____

Food group: _____

Recommended
servings per day: _____

Food group: _____

Recommended
servings per day: _____

Food group: _____

Recommended
servings per day: _____

Food group: _____

Recommended
servings per day: _____

Food group: _____

Recommended
servings per day: _____

2. Complete the following exercises, providing suggestions for improving the diets of the Jones family, James, and Maria (discussed in worksheet 2, "Help! You're the Doctor").

   a. Using the Food Guide Pyramid, create an afternoon snack menu for the Jones family for the next school week. Refer to worksheet #2 to see what they need.

   Monday _____

   Tuesday _____

   Wednesday _____

   Thursday _____

   Friday _____

   b. Suggest drinks and snacks that would help James eat from the one food group he is missing. This group also provides him with calcium, which is good for his bones and teeth.

   _____

   _____

   _____

   _____

   c. List some fun activities that James could do during the week to keep him active. Pick a different activity for each day of the week:

   Sunday _____

   Monday _____

   Tuesday _____

   Wednesday _____

   Thursday _____

   Friday _____

   Saturday_____

   d. Suggest some high-carbohydrate foods, including whole grains, that are low-fat and low in added sugar that Maria should consider eating before playing basketball.

   _____

   _____

   _____

   _____

Solutions

Worksheet 2   Help! You're the Doctor

1. Members of the Jones family have been told by a doctor that they should eat more foods that contain a lot of vitamins and minerals. The family eats a lot of foods from the grain, dairy, and protein food groups, but they obviously need a greater variety of foods in their daily diet.

    List some foods that would help the Jones family improve their diet. List five foods that contain a lot of vitamins and minerals.

    Answer: The Jones family needs to eat more fruits and vegetables. Fruits and vegetables are a wonderful source of vitamins and minerals.

2. James, a fifth-grade student, eats toast for breakfast and a meat sandwich for lunch. He eats an apple or orange each day, and always has some vegetables for his evening meal along with meat, chicken, or fish. He goes to the park or beach with his family on weekends, but during the week his only exercise is walking 150 yards from his home to his school.

    Which food group(s) is missing from James's diet? Why is this food group important? What else could James do to improve his health?

    Answer: James should add foods from the dairy group to his diet. Dairy products provide the calcium his body needs to maintain strong bones and teeth. James would also benefit from more exercise.

3. Maria plays basketball for two hours each afternoon at the school gym. Recently she noticed that she has no energy after the first hour, which is something that never used to happen. She has been watching a lot of television and reading books late at night, and wakes up at 6 A.M. each morning to go to school.

    List three reasons Maria may not have enough energy. How can she improve her energy level?

    Answer: The reason(s) Maria has no energy to play basketball for more than an hour is most likely a combination of factors. By staying up late and waking early, Maria is not getting enough sleep, which makes her feel tired and less energetic. In addition, she may not be eating foods that provide her body with energy, such as high-carbohydrate foods. High-carbohydrate foods can be found in all groups of the Food Guide Pyramid.

Solutions

Worksheet 3   Pyramid Planning

1. The following is the Food Guide Pyramid with the suggested amount of servings for each group:

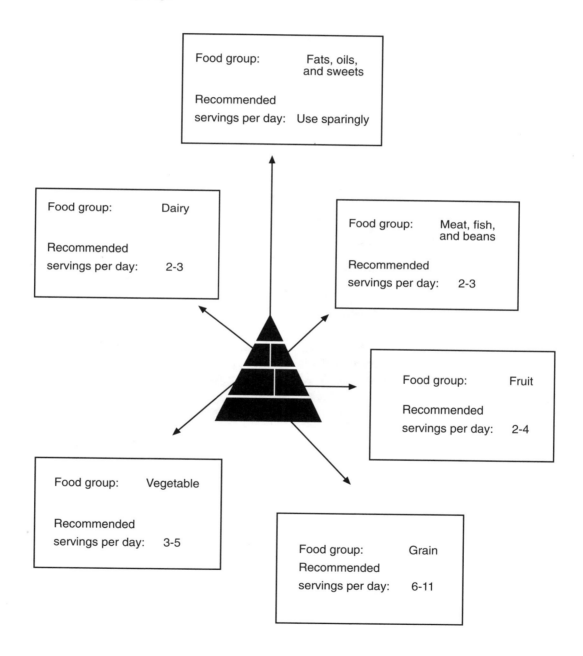

Food group: Fats, oils, and sweets

Recommended
servings per day: Use sparingly

Food group: Dairy

Recommended
servings per day: 2-3

Food group: Meat, fish, and beans

Recommended
servings per day: 2-3

Food group: Fruit

Recommended
servings per day: 2-4

Food group: Vegetable

Recommended
servings per day: 3-5

Food group: Grain
Recommended
servings per day: 6-11

2. Improving the diets of the Jones family, James, and Maria.
   a. Sample snack menu

      Monday: raw carrots with spinach dip

      Tuesday: orange/cantaloupe

      Wednesday: melon with yogurt

      Thursday: raw broccoli with low-fat dip

      Friday: apricot/mango

   b. Drink and snack suggestions for James

      Glass of low-fat milk

      Low-fat cheese

      Broccoli with low-calorie dip

      Whole grain cereal with low-fat milk

      Low-fat yogurt

      Fruit smoothie made with low-fat yogurt

   c. Fun activities for James

      Sunday: basketball

      Monday: roller skating

      Tuesday: bike riding

      Wednesday: baseball

      Thursday: Frisbee

      Friday: jumping rope

      Saturday: soccer

   d. Examples of snack foods that are high in carbohydrates, low-fat, and convenient: mangoes, oranges, pears, plums, grapes, blackberries, apples, figs, fig bars, bread sticks, whole grain toast with jam, whole grain cereal, 100% juice, low-fat milk, whole grain crackers, English muffins, and pretzels.

Teacher Resource Page #1

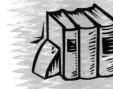

Carbohydrate Foods

Foods that are good sources of carbohydrates:

Baked potato

Banana

Black beans

Black-eyed peas

Brown rice

Corn

Cornflakes

Couscous

Cream of wheat

French bread

Garbanzo beans

Grapes

Green beans

Lima beans

Linguini/macaroni

Low-fat milk

Low-fat yogurt

Mangoes

Mashed potatoes

Navy beans

Nectarines

Oatmeal

Oatmeal raisin cookies

Orange juice

Oranges

Pancakes

Peaches

Pears

Pinto beans

Plantains

Plums

Polenta

Pretzels

Raisin bread

Rice

Spaghetti

Squash

Sweet potatoes

Waffles

Whole grain cereal

Whole wheat bread

Teacher Resource Page #2

Low-Carbohydrate Foods

Examples of foods that are *not* high in carbohydrates:

Meat	Fish
Hamburger (without bun)	Eggs
Hot dog (without bun)	Cucumbers
Cheese	Mushrooms
Lettuce	Greens
Celery	Nuts
Chicken	

Keeping the Balance

Background*

The Food Guide Pyramid provides an excellent example of how to eat a balanced diet every day. If a person chooses the minimum number of servings from each of the five food groups, he or she should be getting most, if not all, of the nutrients needed to maintain good health.

A balanced diet is important because different foods contain different combinations of important nutrients. No single food can supply all the nutrients one needs to maintain good health. This is why balance and variety go hand-in-hand. For example, oranges provide vitamin C, but no vitamin B_{12}; cheese provides vitamin B_{12}, but no vitamin C. It is important to remember that foods in one food group cannot replace those in another. Choosing a variety of foods between groups and within groups will help make your diet more interesting, as well as balanced.

The carbohydrates, fats, and proteins in food supply energy, which is measured in calories. Carbohydrates and proteins provide four calories per gram. Fat contributes more than twice as much—nine calories per gram. Foods that are high in fat are also high in calories.

In order to stay at the same body weight, people must balance the amount of energy in food eaten with the amount of energy the body uses. Achieving this balance doesn't need to occur absolutely every day, but should be achieved generally, such as over a few day's time.

Physical activity is an important way to use up food energy. Most Americans spend much of their working day in activities that require little energy. In addition, many Americans of all ages now spend a lot of leisure time each day being inactive—e.g., watching television or playing computer or video games. To use up dietary energy, people must spend less time doing sedentary activities like sitting and spend more time doing activities like walking to the store or around the block and climbing stairs rather than using elevators. Less sedentary activity and more vigorous activity may help reduce body fat and disease risks.

The kinds and amounts of food people eat affect their ability to maintain weight. High-fat foods contain more calories per serving than other foods and may increase the likelihood of weight gain. However, even when people eat less high-fat food, they still can gain weight from eating too much of foods high in starch, sugar, or protein. Choose sensible portion sizes. Eat a variety of foods. Fruits, vegetables, pasta, rice, bread, and other whole-grain foods are filling but are lower in calories than foods rich in fats or oils.

The pattern of eating may also be important. Snacks provide a large percentage of daily calories for many Americans. Unless nutritious snacks are part of the daily meal plan, snacking may lead to weight gain.

Children need enough food for proper growth. To promote growth and development and prevent obesity, teach children to eat whole grains, vegetables, and fruits, as well as low-fat dairy and other protein-rich foods, and to participate in vigorous activity. Limiting television time and encouraging children to play actively in a safe environment are helpful steps. Although limiting fat intake may help to prevent excess weight gain in children, fat should not be restricted for children younger than two years of age.

* Source of background material: Dietary Guidelines for Americans, 2000.

Estimated Teaching Time and Related Subject Areas

Estimated teaching time: 1 hour

Related subject areas: math, science

Objectives

1. Students will discuss the importance of a balanced diet containing all six types of nutrients.
2. Students will learn ways to balance, over the long term, the food they eat with physical activity.

Materials

1. Transparency #1, "Food, Nutrients, and You"
2. Transparency #2, "Energy Balance"
3. Worksheet #1, "Keeping the Balancing"
4. Worksheet #2, "How is My Balance?"
5. Solutions to worksheet #1
6. Clear drinking glass
7. Pitcher of water (add food coloring for visibility)
8. Low-sided baking dish

Procedure

Part I

1. Set up the following demonstration so all students can see it. Place the drinking glass in the baking dish (to catch any overflow of water) and fill the glass to the very top with colored water. Explain that this full glass represents a person who is full of the nutrients needed to remain healthy and active.
2. Ask the students what happens to the level of nutrients in the person's body throughout the day. (The level goes down.) Pour some of the water back into the pitcher to show a partly empty glass.
3. Ask the students what the person needs to do to get back to the right level of nutrients. (Eat nutritious foods.) Fill the glass up to the top again.
4. Ask the students what happens when a person regularly eats more than he/she needs for her/his daily energy requirements for growth and maintenance of body functions. (He/she will put on weight.) Pour extra water into the already full glass, allowing it to overflow. Explain that the overflowing water represents extra energy that our bodies will need to store, usually in the form of extra fat.
5. Explain to the class that in today's lesson they will take a closer look at how they can get nutrients their bodies need without getting too many calories beyond their requirements for growth and maintenance.

Part II

1. Ask the students this question: "What are nutrients and why are they important to a person?" The following definition may be helpful: "Nutrients are the parts of foods your body uses to grow, repair itself, and give you energy."
2. Project transparency #1, "Food, Nutrients, and You," and discuss the six types of nutrients, their functions, and the food sources where they may be found. Explain

that it is important to eat a variety of foods in order to get all of the nutrients the body needs.

You may want to make an extra laminated copy of the "Food, Nutrients, and You" transparency and create a game that allows students to review the contents of the worksheet.

3. Write the word "calorie" on the board. Explain that a calorie is a measure of how much energy a food gives you. Some foods, such as fruits and vegetables, are full of nutrients, and are also low in calories. Other foods, such as "junk foods," can have many calories and very few nutrients.

   Tell the students, "If a food contains 100 calories, it gives you 100 units of energy. Most adults need 1,500 to 2,200 calories a day, depending on how much they exercise. You are still growing, and that requires energy, so you probably need about 2,000-3,000 calories a day, depending on how physically active you are."

4. Project "Energy Balance," transparency #2, and explain that if the nutrients and calories taken into the body and the energy used by the body are not equal, the body can have problems. Point to the top picture and ask, "What can happen if the nutrients and energy used are greater than the nutrients and calories taken in?" (Answer: The body gets tired, can't grow or repair tissue, begins to break down lean body tissue and fat stores, loses weight.) Ask, "What could a person do to fix the imbalance?" (Answer: Eat more nutrients and calories.)

5. Point to the middle picture and ask, "What might happen if the amount of calories taken in is consistently greater than the amount of energy used?" (Answer: Excess energy will be stored as fat, and the body will put on weight.) Ask, "What could this person do to fix the imbalance?" (Answer: Eat fewer calories; exercise more.)

6. Point to the bottom picture and explain that eating the right amount of nutrients and calories for a person's size and activity level means the body creates an energy and nutrient balance. This is the way to maintain a healthy body.

7. Have the students form pairs and distribute the "Keeping the Balance" worksheet. Explain that everything a person does, even sleeping, requires the body to use calories for energy. Some activities require a lot more units of energy than others. The chart shows approximately how many calories are required for a 100-pound person doing various activities. Instruct each student to use the chart and his or her own knowledge to answer the questions on the worksheet.

8. Once the students have completed the worksheet, discuss their answers. Encourage them to think about how they might use this information to improve their own energy balance.

9. (optional) Distribute the "How Is My Balance?" worksheet and have students fill it out for a day. You may want to repeat this activity more than once.

Food, Nutrients, and You

Table 14.1   Food, Nutrients, and You

Nutrient & Functions	Food Sources
Water	
• Helps cool your body when it's working hard	Water, drinks without caffeine, fruit, soup
• Helps you digest your food	
• Helps nutrients get to different parts of the body	
Carbohydrates	
• Give you energy	Whole grains, fruit, starchy & root vegetables (like potatoes, yams, & sweet potatoes)
• Can be stored as energy for later use	
• Give sweetness and texture to foods	
• Provide a good source of vitamins, minerals, and fiber	
Minerals	
• Help your blood carry oxygen and nutrients to your muscles and other body parts	Whole grains, lean meat, milk, vegetables, fruit, cheese, legumes (dry beans)
• Help build strong bones and teeth	
Protein	
• Builds and repairs muscles	Meat, poultry, fish, dry beans, nuts, milk & milk products, eggs, tofu
• Helps your body grow	
Vitamins	
• Help you to see better at night	Vegetables, fruit, fish, whole grains, milk & milk products
• Help your body get energy from the food you eat	
• Help your body heal cuts and bruises	
• Help you fight off infections	
Fat	
• Gives you energy, especially for long-term use	Vegetable oil, meats & nuts, milk products (cheese)
• Makes you feel less hungry	
• Makes food taste good	
• Helps keep your skin smooth	

Energy Balance

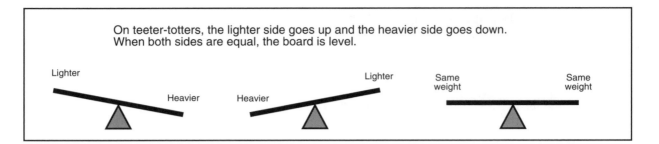

On teeter-totters, the lighter side goes up and the heavier side goes down.
When both sides are equal, the board is level.

Lighter

Heavier

Heavier

Lighter

Same weight

Same weight

Not enough nutrients and calories

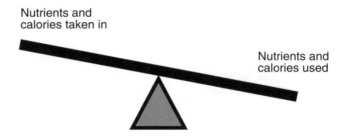

Nutrients and calories taken in

Nutrients and calories used

Too many nutrients and calories

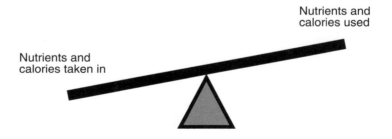

Nutrients and calories used

Nutrients and calories taken in

Nutrient balance

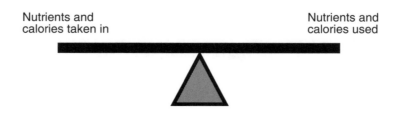

Nutrients and calories taken in

Nutrients and calories used

Keeping the Balance

| Everything you do, even sleeping and growing, requires your body to use calories. | | Almost everything you eat or drink, except water, contains calories. |

Activity	Calories used in 1/2 hour by a 100-lb. person
bike riding	93
running	183
swimming	150
resting/sitting	40
walking	81

1. How many calories would you use watching television from 4:00 to 6:30 P.M.?

_____

2a. How many more calories would you use if you rode your bike for an hour compared to if you watched TV for an hour?

_____

2b. How many extra calories would you use over the course of a week if you substituted an hour of bike riding for an hour of TV watching each day?

_____

2c. How about for a month (30 days)?

_____

3. Jason spends the day in school, then takes the bus home. He fixes himself a snack (usually chips and a soda), then does his homework. After dinner, Jason is allowed one and one-half hours of television or computer games. He sometimes reads a book or talks with friends on the phone. Jason is a little overweight. What can he do to improve his weight and overall health?

_____

4. How many calories would you use if you ran laps around the playground for 10 minutes, then rode your bicycle home for 10 minutes?

_____

5. *Extra Credit:* Assume you weigh 100 pounds. How many calories would you use walking 20 minutes to your friend's house and 20 minutes back each day?

_____

How Is My Balance?

Name _____ Date _____

Draw a picture of the scale to show how you think you balanced your nutrients and calories with the energy you used today. (Remember: Growing takes energy too, probably less than 100 calories a day.)

Here are the changes I want to make tomorrow to create a better nutrition/energy balance:

_____

_____

_____

_____

_____

_____

Solutions

Worksheet 1   Keeping the Balance

1. How many calories would you use watching television from 4:00 to 6:30 P.M.?
    Answer:

    Step 1: resting/sitting = 40 calories/30 minutes

    Step 2: 4:00 P.M.-6:30 P.M. = 2.5 hours or five 30-minute periods

    Step 3: 5 (30-minute periods) × 40 calories/30 minutes = 200 calories

2a. How many more calories would you use if you rode your bike for an hour compared to if you watched TV for an hour?
    Answer:

    Step 1: 186 calories – 80 calories = 106 calories

2b. How many extra calories would you use over the course of a week if you substituted an hour of bike riding for an hour of TV watching each day?
    Answer:

    Step 1: 106 calories/day × 7 days = 742 calories

2c. How about for a month (30 days)?
    Answer:

    Step 1: 106 calories/day × 30 days = 3,180 calories

3. Jason spends the day in school, then takes the bus home. He fixes himself a snack (usually chips and a soda), then does his homework. After dinner, Jason is allowed one and one-half hours of television or computer games. He sometimes reads a book or talks with friends on the phone. Jason is a little overweight. What can he do to improve his weight and overall health?
    Possible answers:

    Jason could walk or ride his bike to school.

    Jason could do something active in the evening.

    Jason could eat fruit instead of chips and soda.

4. How many calories would you use if you ran laps around the playground for 10 minutes, then rode your bicycle home (10 minutes)?
    Answer:

    Step 1: (183 calories/half hour of running) ÷ (3 10-minute periods in a half hour) = 61 calories for each 10-minute period running

    Step 2: (93 calories/half hour of bike riding) ÷ (3 10-minute periods in a half hour) = 31 calories for each 10-minute period of bike riding

    Step 3: 61 calories for 10 minutes of running + 31 calories for 10 minutes of riding bike = 92 calories

5. *Extra Credit:* Assume you weigh 100 pounds. How many calories would you use walking 20 minutes to your friend's house and 20 minutes back each day?

Answer:

Step 1: Walking 20 minutes to friend's house + 20 minutes home = 40 minutes of walking, or 4 10-minute periods

Step 2: (81 calories/half hour of walking) ÷ (3 10-minute periods in a half hour) = 27 calories for every 10 minutes of walking

Step 3: (27 calories for every 10 minutes of walking) × (4 10-minute periods of walking) = 108 calories

The Safe Workout: A Review

Background

The human body can do amazing things. However, in order for the body to perform well, it must be taken care of. It is important to choose good foods, to exercise regularly, to stay away from harmful substances (such as tobacco and drugs), and to get plenty of sleep to keep the body healthy. The body needs good food to give it energy, to help it grow, and to repair itself. Exercising regularly also helps keep the body healthy. Some exercises make the heart, lungs, and blood vessels stronger. Some exercises help with flexibility and the body's ability to bend. Some exercises help maintain a healthy weight. The body needs all kinds of exercise. This lesson will teach students the safe way to exercise and at the same time review the Food Guide Pyramid.

This lesson reviews the five parts of a safe workout. The concept of the safe workout is introduced in lesson 3 of the grade 4 lesson-set, which includes a detailed description of the different workout components. The amount of time spent reviewing the components in this lesson will depend on student exposure to the safe workout the previous year when they were in fourth grade.

The five parts of the safe workout are important to help prevent injuries while exercising. These five parts are (1) the warm-up, (2) the stretch, (3) the fitness activity, (4) the cool-down, and (5) the cool-down stretch. Each part will be introduced by stating why it is important and how to do it correctly. Because of time constraints, the parts of the lesson workout are shorter than what they normally should be in an actual workout. For example, the lesson warm-up is only one to two minutes long, when ideally the warm-up should be at least five minutes. What's important is that the students learn that a warm-up is the first part of a safe workout and that it should be done at home before they exercise on their bike or play basketball.

Exercising and doing the five parts of a safe workout is only half of the story! In addition to being physically active, eating right is the other half of the winning combination that keeps our bodies healthy. The students will be learning about the Food Guide Pyramid while moving!

This activity can be used as a practice lesson for the other physical activity lessons, which will be done in the gymnasium, community room, or cafeteria.

Estimated Teaching Time and Related Subject Area

Estimated teaching time: 1 hour, 20 minutes

Related subject area: physical education

Objectives

Students will be able to

1. identify and sequence the components of a safe and healthy workout,

2. discuss and demonstrate each component of a safe workout,

3. identify the components of the Food Guide Pyramid and how to make daily food choices based on the Food Guide Pyramid recommendations, and

4. choose positive health practices based on knowledge from the safe workout and the Food Guide Pyramid.

Materials

1. Pictures of various foods
2. Food Guide Pyramid poster
3. Stretching and Strength Fitness diagrams (see appendix, pp. 453-459)
4. Teacher Resource Page #1, "What Counts As a Serving?"

Procedure

1. Go over pertinent vocabulary for the lesson.

   Warm-up: the first part of the safe workout, in which slow movements get the body ready for stretching and the fitness activity

   Stretch: the part of the safe workout in which you do exercises that improve flexibility fitness and get the body ready for fitness activity

   Fitness activity: the part of the safe workout in which strength and endurance fitness exercises are performed

   Cool-down: the part of the safe workout in which your body slows down and recovers from the fitness activity

   Cool-down stretch: the last part of the safe workout in which you do exercises that improve flexibility fitness

   Pacing: maintaining a comfortable speed so that you can perform your exercise over an extended period of time

   Flexibility fitness: ability to bend; the part of fitness that stretches the muscles and areas around the muscles to get your body ready for action

   Strength fitness: the part of fitness that makes your muscles (except the heart muscle) stronger and healthier

   Endurance fitness: the part of fitness that helps improve the heart muscle, lungs, and blood vessels, and helps maintain weight

2. Provide motivation for the lesson. Ask students to raise their hands if they would like to

   • grow up to be as healthy as they can be,

   • be able to play, dance, and run longer, and

   • feel good about themselves.

   Tell students that if they raised their hands to any of the above questions, then this lesson is an important one for them. It's their chance to learn the benefits and importance of eating right and exercising.

3. Provide a mini-introduction to the lesson.

   "We learned that it is important for our bodies to get the right amounts and kinds of food every day. We also learned that we should eat a variety of different foods and that we should eat foods from all of the different groups that are represented in the Food Guide Pyramid. The pyramid is a guide to help us learn to eat foods that will help our bodies stay healthy, grow, and perform physical activities such as playing and dancing. Regular, moderate to vigorous physical activity is also important to our body's health.

"Just as the Food Guide Pyramid steers us in the right direction so that we eat foods that make us healthy, the safe workout steers us in the right direction so that we exercise and participate in physical activities in ways that are good for our bodies."

4. Have the class form five groups and assign each group one of the five food groups from the Food Guide Pyramid: group 1—grain group; group 2—vegetable group; group 3—fruit group; group 4—meat group; group 5—dairy group. Tell students that you (the teacher) represent the tip of the pyramid—fats, oils, and sweets.

5. Review with the class the foods that belong to each group. Have each group work together to create a list of as many foods as they can that belong to their group. Have each group share their list with the class and see if the other groups can add any additional foods.

6. After each group has shared its list, review the recommended servings per day for each group (grains: 6-11; vegetables: 3-5; fruit: 2-4; dairy: 2-3; meat, beans and fish: 2-3).

7. Keep the students in their food groups. Stress that to be healthy and energized, keeping their bodies moving (through exercise) is just as important as eating right. The following description covers all five areas of the safe workout including the shopping fitness activity, which is a movement game that reviews the Food Guide Pyramid and the recommended number of servings per day of each food group. In addition, the Stay Healthy Corner, where we review what we have learned and how we can apply it to our daily lives, will be covered.

1. The warm-up (1-2 minutes)

2. The stretch (1-2 minutes)

3. The fitness activity (15-20 minutes)

4. The cool-down (1 minute)

5. The cool-down stretch (1 minute)

6. The Stay Healthy Corner (4-5 minutes)

The Warm-Up: 1-2 Minutes

Why Warm Up?

- Helps prevent injuries.
- Increases body temperature; gets body warmer before you make it work hard.
- Gets body ready for the rest of the workout including the stretching and fitness activity.

How to Warm Up

- Perform a series of slow movements—e.g., slow jogging in place, slow jumping jacks.

What to Emphasize

- Car analogy: your body is like a cold car—warm it up and then move it!
- If you do not warm up, you are more likely to get injured.
- You should always warm up before exercising, even when you are at home.
- Always do the movements very slowly to warm up.
- For example, for a bike ride, warm up by riding slowly at first.
- Likewise, when throwing a ball, throw slowly at first.

Examples of Student Warm-Up Formations

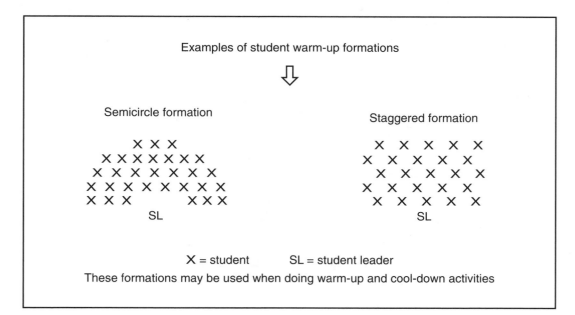

Examples of student warm-up formations

Semicircle Formation

1. Students should establish and maintain a safe distance between those students who are in front of, in back of, and on either side of themselves.
2. There should be enough room between students so that they will be able to do all stretches and exercises without fear of inadvertently hitting or being hit by another student.

   Students should stand so they are facing you and/or the group leader. Likewise, they should be spaced so there is not another student directly in front of them.

Staggered Formation

1. Have a group of five students form a row with enough space so that they cannot touch each other if their arms are extended at shoulder height. Five more students will form a second row behind row one. Students in the second row should stand behind and between the two students in the row in front of them and, like those in the first row, should make sure that there is enough space between them. Continue to put students in rows until all have been placed.
2. Students should stand so that they are facing (and can see) you and/or the student leader who will be in front of the room.

The Stretch: 1-2 Minutes

Why Stretch?

- Improves flexibility fitness: the ability to bend, twist, and stretch; the ability of muscles and joints to move in their complete range of motion.
- Muscles can work better when they are long and bendable.
- Body can move better; better at sport skills.
- Helps prevent injuries.

How to Stretch

- Hold stretch for 10 or more seconds (count out loud: 1 Mississippi, 2 Mississippi . . . to 10 Mississippi).
- Don't bounce; hold stretch gently.
- Stretch slowly.
- Use proper form to avoid injuries.
- Examples of stretches are neck stretch, butterfly, and quad burner (thigh stretch).

Examples of Student Stretches

Have students perform stretches as they appear in the diagrams in the appendix (pp. 453-456). One student or a small group of students can help demonstrate the stretches for the class.

What to Emphasize

- Stretching improves flexibility fitness.
- Activities such as riding a bike or doing push-ups do not improve flexibility.
- Even if you aren't going to be doing a fitness activity, stretch at home while watching TV or when doing nothing in particular.
- Hold stretches for 10 or more seconds.
- Use slow movements; don't bounce.

The Fitness Activity: 15-20 Minutes

Why Endurance Fitness?

- Helps improve health of heart, lung, and blood vessels (cardiovascular fitness).
- Helps maintain a healthy weight.
- Gives you energy.

How to Improve Endurance Fitness

- Do activities that involve nonstop, continuous movement, e.g., nonstop bike riding, nonstop walking, nonstop rope jumping (students may jog or walk in place to demonstrate endurance activities in class).
- Find a pace (speed) you can do for a long time—"Pace, don't race!"
- As a goal, do endurance activities three to four days a week for 20-30 minutes.
- Find an endurance activity you like so you will want to do it.

What to Emphasize

- Pace, don't race.
- Getting fit should be fun.

Endurance Activity Game #1

Eat Well & *Keep Moving*: Making a Healthful Menu Game

a. Equipment needed
   1. Food models for general audiences (a variety of food pictures from the different food groups)

    2. Five hula hoops or boxes

    3. Music to move to (optional)

b. Introduction

Explain to students, "The purpose of the game is to determine if each of you knows which food items from the Food Guide Pyramid fit correctly into your food group. We are also playing this game so that we can improve fitness and learn how to pace ourselves so that we can make our bodies stronger. Making our bodies stronger will enable us to do an activity for longer periods of time without becoming tired."

c. Instructions

1. Keep class in their five food groups and ask each group to form a line (see "Gym Line Formation for Shopping Fitness Activities"). The formation used can depend upon the layout and space of the room.

2. Explain the path the students will take so that there is no confusion and students can perform the tasks safely.

3. Using a cone or distinguishable line, designate a place where the first person in each line can stand. The second person in line will move to this place after the first student has left the position.

4. Place a hula hoop to the right of each line of students (refer to diagram "Gym Line Formation for Shopping Fitness Activities"). This hula hoop can be called a plate or a refrigerator. Each student will place the food that he/she collects in this area and then jog to the back of his/her food group line. Explain to students,

   "The area inside the basketball key (or similar area) has pictures of food all over the floor and is called the grocery store. Each of you will go shopping for a food that is found in your food group. The first person in each group will jog in a straight path until he or she gets to the grocery store area. Once there, select the correct food for your group, pick it up, and jog back to the plate/refrigerator (hula hoop) and deposit the food picture in it. After this, jog to the back of your line and jog in place until every member of every group has completed this task at least once.

   "This is not a race or a competition between groups."

5. This activity will begin with the teacher saying, "Let's go shopping for food!" The entire class will jog lightly in place until the last student in each food group has had a turn and has taken a place at the end of the line.

6. As the first students in each line are performing this activity, coach them by reminding them to come back on their path so that they can safely jog to their plate/refrigerator.

7. As the game progresses, tell the students to "Pace, don't race," so they can continue jogging until each member of their group has gone shopping and brought a food item back. Remind the next people in line to wait until the jogger has arrived at the end of the line before starting out so that the activity can be done safely.

   After the first group of students has gone through the course and has moved to the back of the line, ask if there are any questions. If there are no questions, tell the students that they are about to begin with the set of students who are now first in line.

8. Once each group has collected at least 11 food pictures, have each group sit around their pictures and make sure all of the foods they collected belong in their food group. If they think that a food is in the wrong food group, have one of the students bring it back to the food area.

9. As a class, review the food choices each group made. When all food groups are satisfied with their choices, review the recommended servings per day for each food group.

10. Have each group choose a number of food pictures that falls within the range of the recommended number of servings per day for their food group (e.g., grains group will pick 6-11 food pictures).

11. Bring the class together with their choices and talk about what a serving size would be for some of the foods they picked (see Teacher Resource Page #1, "What Counts As a Serving?"). Stress that while it is important to eat from all of the food groups, it is also important to know about serving size. Knowing what the serving sizes are and following the Food Guide Pyramid's recommended number of servings for each group means we won't eat too much or too little of any kind of food. This is important because we need the nutrients found in foods—protein, carbohydrates, fat, minerals, and vitamins—to help us grow, give us energy, and repair our bodies if needed. What we have to strive for is *moderation* and not eating too much or too little of any food group. Explain to students that "Eating Right and Exercising are *best friends*!" We need to eat healthfully and exercise too! This is why the fitness activity combines exercise with learning about the Food Guide Pyramid and the recommended number of servings each day.

12. Tell the students it is time for the cool-down. Ask students to walk around the gymnasium, cafeteria, or community room three times, with everyone moving in the same direction.

The Cool-Down: 1 Minute

What to Emphasize

- Move slowly.
- Remember to cool down after exercising at home too.

The Cool-Down Stretch: 1 Minute

Why the Cool-Down Stretch?

- Helps prevent soreness.
- Improves flexibility fitness.

How to Do the Cool-Down Stretch

Examples are butterfly, triceps stretch, thigh stretch.

What to Emphasize

- Stretching improves flexibility fitness.
- Activities such as riding a bike or doing push-ups do not improve flexibility.
- Even if you aren't going to be doing a fitness activity, stretch at home while watching TV or when doing nothing in particular.
- Hold stretches for 10 or more seconds.
- Use slow movements; don't bounce.

The Stay Healthy Corner: 4-5 Minutes

1. When the cool-down stretch has been completed, have all the groups reassemble.

2. Allow each group several minutes to verbally share their food choices and servings per day with the class.

3. Talk about how they can practice using this healthy eating information at home. Ask students what kind of movement and exercises they can do at home with their family and friends. Stress to them that having the family involved is very helpful. Let students know that this involvement begins at the grocery store. Ask students what they can do to help get their family more involved with healthy lifestyles.

Gym line formation
for shopping fitness activities

[**X** = one student, □ = teacher (fats, oils, and sweets)]

The purpose of the game is to determine if each student in a group knows which food items from the Food Guide Pyramid fit into their food group. We are also playing this game so that we can become fit and learn how to pace ourselves so that we can make our bodies stronger and able to do an activity for a certain length of time without becoming tired.

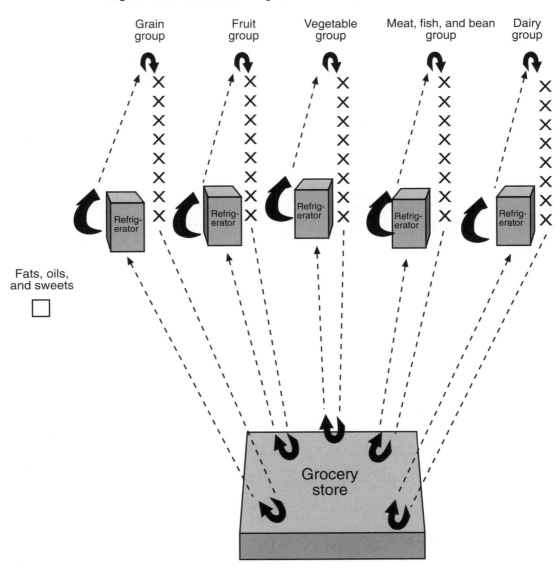

Classroom Line Formation Options

The best option depends on the layout of the classroom

Option #1

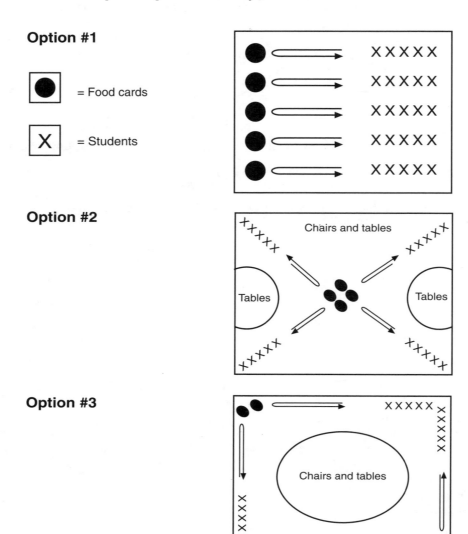

= Food cards

= Students

Option #2

Option #3

Teacher Resource Page #1

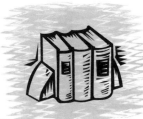

What Counts As a Serving?

- **Grains group (especially whole grain bread, cereal, rice, and pasta):** 1 slice whole grain bread; 3/4 cup dry cereal; 1/2 cup cooked cereal, rice, or pasta; 1/2 English muffin, 1/2 hamburger bun, or 1/2 bagel; 1 roll or medium-sized muffin
- **Vegetable group:** 1 cup raw, leafy vegetables; 1/2 cup other cooked or chopped vegetables; 3/4 cup vegetable juice
- **Fruit group:** 1 medium apple, banana, orange; 1/2 cup cooked, chopped, or canned fruit; 3/4 cup fruit juice; 1/4 cup dried fruit; 1/2 grapefruit; 1/4 cantaloupe
- **Milk, yogurt, and cheese group:** 1 cup milk or yogurt; 1.5 oz. natural cheese; 2 oz. processed cheese; 1/2 cup cottage cheese
- **Dry beans, eggs, nuts, fish, and meat and poultry group:** 2-3 oz. cooked lean meat, poultry, or fish; 1/2 cup cooked beans; 1 egg; 2 tablespoons peanut butter; 1/4 cup nuts or seeds

For combination foods, such as pizza, estimate the food group servings for each group—bread, milk, vegetable, meat, etc. For example, two slices of vegetable pizza may equal one serving of dairy (from the cheese), two servings of grain (from the crust), and one serving of vegetables (from the tomato sauce and vegetable toppings).

Hunting for Hidden Fat

Background

Fat is an important part of our diets. Fat helps in the absorption and transport of fat-soluble vitamins such as vitamins A, D, E, and K. Fat is the primary way energy is stored in the body, and it also makes foods taste good. In addition, some fats (which come from plant sources) are essential for healthy skin and hair.

The problem is that most Americans consume too much of the wrong type of fat. This is thought to be the reason that so many people die or are disabled by heart attacks. Every year over half a million people die in this country from heart disease; heart disease is the leading cause of early death and disability in the United States. Many studies have shown a strong relationship between heart disease and high intake of saturated and *trans* fats. The good news is that if we decrease the dietary fat, we can reduce our risk of heart disease.

Saturated fat

Saturated fat (for example, butter or lard) tends to be a solid at room temperature and comes primarily from animal sources (meat and dairy); high intake of saturated fats increases the risk for heart disease. Foods high in saturated fat tend to raise blood cholesterol.

Unsaturated fat

Unsaturated fat (fat that is usually liquid at room temperature), such as vegetable oil or olive oil, decreases the risk for heart disease. Unsaturated or liquid fat can be converted to *trans* fat or more solid forms through a process called hydrogenation. Margarine, for example, is made by hydrogenating a liquid oil, such as soybean oil, until it becomes more saturated and remains solid at room temperature. There is growing evidence that hydrogenated fat (a major source of *trans* fat) found in high amounts in stick margarine may also increase the risk of heart disease.

Cholesterol

The body makes the cholesterol it requires. Cholesterol also is obtained from food. Dietary cholesterol comes from animal sources such as egg yolks, meat (especially organ meats such as liver), poultry, fish, and higher-fat milk products. Many of these foods are also high in saturated fats. Choosing foods with less cholesterol and with less *trans* and saturated fats will help lower your blood cholesterol levels. The Nutrition Facts Label lists the Daily Value for cholesterol as 300 mg. You can keep your cholesterol intake at this level or lower by eating more grain products, vegetables, and fruits, and by limiting intake of foods that contain cholesterol.

Trans fat

Trans fat is produced during the hydrogenation of vegetable oils. Hydrogenation hardens oils to make them spreadable (e.g., margarine) and improves shelf life. However, *trans* fat raises the body's LDL level (commonly known as the "bad" cholesterol) and lowers the HDL levels (the "good" cholesterol). In a typical American diet, *trans* fat is found mostly in foods that contain hydrogenated or partially hydrogenated vegetable oils, particularly in baked goods such as cookies and crackers. If hydrogenated or partially hydrogenated oil is used, it will be listed in the ingredient list on the food package. *Trans* fat is also found in animal fat.

The Food Guide Pyramid is designed to limit daily fat intake to no more than 30 percent of total calories from fat. A diet low in saturated and *trans* fat may reduce your risk for heart disease and could also help you maintain a healthy body weight. This is the reason some of the foods in the three food groups near the top of the pyramid should be consumed in smaller quantities. These foods—dairy foods, animal meats, and processed or fried foods—tend to contain a lot more saturated and *trans* fats than other foods in the pyramid.

However, within each of these food groups, there are lower-fat options from which to choose. Low-fat or nonfat milk, yogurt, and cheeses are now available in supermarkets; while fish, poultry without skin, and dried beans provide protein without a lot of saturated fat. Foods in the "fats, sweets, and oils" food group at the very top of the pyramid are meant to be consumed in small quantities and relatively infrequently. A lot of foods we call "junk" foods fit into this food group. They tend to be very high in salt and in fat (especially saturated and *trans* fats) and low in the nutrients that help decrease the risk of infection or disease.

Teacher Information: How is % Daily Value for Fat Calculated?

Although all food labels provide %DV for nutrients, the following describes how the % Daily Value for one specific nutrient (fat) is calculated.

For a particular food, divide the number of grams of fat per serving by 65. Sixty-five (65) is used because it is recommended that a person eating a 2,000-calorie daily diet consume no more than 65 grams of fat each day.

For example: A serving of tuna salad has 14 grams of fat; $14 \div 65 = 22\%$. Therefore a serving of tuna salad contains 22% DV for fat for a person who eats 2,000 calories a day.

Reading food labels is an effective way to compare the fat and nutrient content of various snack foods. The place to find out whether a food is relatively high or low in a nutrient is the % Daily Value column on the Nutrition Facts label on food packages. The % Daily Value for total fat and saturated fat are important. If, for individual foods, the % Daily Value is 5 or less for total fat or saturated fat, the food is considered low-fat (low in total fat or saturated fat). The more foods chosen that have a % Daily Value of 5 or less for total fat and saturated fat, the easier it is to eat a healthier daily diet. The overall daily goal should be to select foods that together do not exceed 100% of the Daily Value for total fat and saturated fat.

The % Daily Value is based on a diet of 2,000 calories per day.

Estimated Teaching Time and Related Subject Areas

Estimated teaching time: 1 hour, 15 minutes

Related subject areas: math, science, art

Objectives

1. Students will explain why fat is an important part of one's diet.
2. Students will discriminate between solid and liquid fat.
3. Students will be able to examine food labels to identify those that contain fats.

Materials

1. Chalkboard
2. Food wrappers (including nutrition labels) of canned fruits and vegetables, soups, candy bar, desserts, baked goods

3. Small container

4. A piece of cotton or a feather

5. Food labels from a variety of foods (ask students to bring from home)

6. Transparency #1, "The Food Guide Pyramid"

7. Transparency #2, "Reading the Food Label"

8. Handout #1, "Food Labels" (Select a sample to copy to round out the collection of labels brought in by students.)

9. Handout #2, "Reading the Food Label"

10. Worksheet #1, "Can You Find It?"

Procedure

Part I

1. Prior to class, place a piece of cotton, paper, or a feather in a small, covered, opaque container.

2. Ask students to guess the contents (provide a few clues). Have them give reasons for their answers.

3. After several guesses have been given, say to students, "Some of the foods we eat are like this container. They contain hidden ingredients that cannot be seen. Today, we're going to go on a 'hunt' for foods that contain fat."

Part II

1. Display transparency #1, "Food Guide Pyramid," and review the recommended number of servings for each food group and identify the group for fats, oils, and sweets with students.

2. Discuss with students the reasons fat is an important part of their diets (see background material).

3. Tell students that they will investigate all of the food groups in the Food Guide Pyramid that can contain fats.

4. Stress the fact that there are different types of fats, and that a person should pay attention to the types (saturated, *trans*, or unsaturated) of fats eaten as well as the total amount of fat eaten. (In 1991, Americans got, on average, about 34% of their calories from fat, while the Dietary Guidelines for Americans recommend no more than 30%.)

Part III

1. Distribute handout #1, "Reading the Food Label," and food labels and/or copies of food labels to students. If possible, be sure there is a wide variety of labels, including canned/frozen fruits and vegetables, desserts, and frozen dinners.

2. Explain to students that food labels contain information that can help a person make smart decisions about whether a particular food fits into the healthful and balanced diet he/she is trying to eat.

3. Display transparency #2 and distribute handout #2 (both are entitled "Reading the Food Label") to students. Explain that one specific thing food labels address is the amount and type (saturated or unsaturated) of fat and cholesterol contained in a food. Food labels also present other information, such as the number of calories a food provides, certain vitamins and minerals a food

contains, and a list of ingredients in the food (with the most abundant ingredient listed first).

4. Name one of the foods for which there is a label, and before examining the label, have students decide if they think the food choice contains fat and saturated fat. Record students' answers on the board before investigations begin.

5. Have students identify the following from each of the food labels and ingredients list:

Food name _____

Serving size_____

Total fat per serving _____

Saturated fat per serving _____

% Daily Value (%DV) of saturated fat_____

% Daily Value (%DV) of total fat _____

Explain that the "% Daily Value of fat" (% DV) number can help them figure out how servings of food contribute to their daily maximum allowance of fat. If they add together the percentages of daily value of fat and saturated fat of all the foods they eat in a day, it should total no more than 100%. Ask for volunteers to stand and state the % Daily Value of total fat found on their food labels. As each student stands, add the percentages until the total reaches 100%. Try different combinations of foods.

6. Write on the board the following words: bacon, steak, chicken, fish, fries. Discuss foods that contain "visible" fats (which can be seen before, during, and after preparation). Examples: bacon, steak, fries, etc. Point out that some foods may not appear to have fats in them, but actually do have fats hidden inside. Identify that the following foods contain hidden fat: chicken with skin, lunch meats, candy bars, hot dogs, pies, cheese, cakes, doughnuts, Twinkies, puddings, ice creams, cookies.

7. Ask students the following question: "What are some foods that you know are prepared with fats/oils?"

Sample responses: French fries, doughnuts, pies, meats, cakes, fried fish, fried chicken, etc.

8. Have students describe the preparation process. As each type of fat (butter, oil, lard, margarine, etc.) is mentioned, list it on the board.

Sample:

What?	How prepared?	Using what?
French fries	Deep fried	Vegetable oil, lard, margarine
Cake	Baked	Butter, oil
Fish	Fried	Vegetable oil, lard
Chicken	Fried	Vegetable oil, lard

9. Have students distinguish between fats that are solid at room temperature and fats that are liquid at room temperature. (Butter, lard, Crisco shortening, and partially hydrogenated vegetable oil are solid at room temperature; most vegetable oils—including olive oil—and squeeze margarine are liquid at room temperature.)

10. Have students tell what happens to solid fat when it is heated. (It becomes liquid.)

11. Explain to students that most of the time they should choose fats that are liquid at room temperature over fats that are solid at room temperature. Liquid fats are better for the body.

12. Distribute worksheet #1, "Can You Find It?" Have students (in pairs or small groups) examine various food labels and ingredient lists (provided) and record the amount of fat and saturated fat in each food selection on the "Can You Find It?" worksheet. Have students make bar graphs to compare the amount of fat in various foods.

Part IV

1. Have students identify the low-saturated fat foods that they should probably eat more of in order to reduce the amount of saturated fat in their diet. Use the activity found on worksheet #1, "Can You Find It?" as a basis for this discussion.

2. Stress that it's OK to eat no more than one small serving each day of high-fat foods (also known as "sometimes" foods). Moderation is the message.

Part V

1. Have students look in their refrigerators and pantries at home and make a list of foods they find that contain less than 5% Daily Value for saturated fat per serving. A food with less than 5% Daily Value for saturated fat per serving is considered a "low-saturated fat" item by the FDA.

2. Have students collect and make a collage of labels from foods with less than 5% Daily Value for saturated fat. Encourage them to be creative in designing their collage and to add a message about nutrition and low-saturated fat foods appropriate for other students in their class or school. Display the collages for others to view.

The Food Guide Pyramid

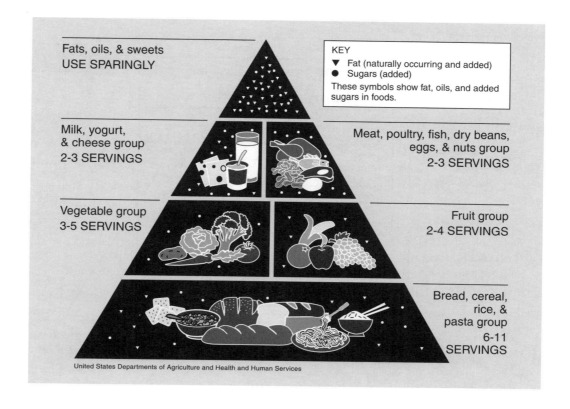

Fats, oils, & sweets
USE SPARINGLY

KEY
▼ Fat (naturally occurring and added)
● Sugars (added)
These symbols show fat, oils, and added sugars in foods.

Milk, yogurt,
& cheese group
2-3 SERVINGS

Meat, poultry, fish, dry beans,
eggs, & nuts group
2-3 SERVINGS

Vegetable group
3-5 SERVINGS

Fruit group
2-4 SERVINGS

Bread, cereal,
rice, &
pasta group
6-11
SERVINGS

United States Departments of Agriculture and Health and Human Services

2 Reading the Food Label

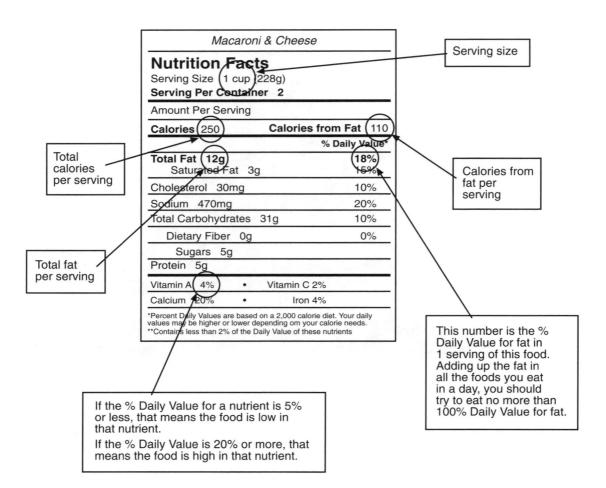

Macaroni & Cheese

Nutrition Facts
Serving Size 1 cup (228g)
Serving Per Container 2

Amount Per Serving

Calories 250   **Calories from Fat** 110

% Daily Value*

Total Fat 12g		**18%**
Saturated Fat 3g		15%
Cholesterol 30mg		10%
Sodium 470mg		20%
Total Carbohydrates 31g		10%
Dietary Fiber 0g		0%
Sugars 5g		
Protein 5g		

Vitamin A 4%	•	Vitamin C 2%
Calcium 20%	•	Iron 4%

*Percent Daily Values are based on a 2,000 calorie diet. Your daily values may be higher or lower depending om your calorie needs.
**Contains less than 2% of the Daily Value of these nutrients

Serving size

Total calories per serving

Calories from fat per serving

Total fat per serving

This number is the % Daily Value for fat in 1 serving of this food. Adding up the fat in all the foods you eat in a day, you should try to eat no more than 100% Daily Value for fat.

If the % Daily Value for a nutrient is 5% or less, that means the food is low in that nutrient.
If the % Daily Value is 20% or more, that means the food is high in that nutrient.

Plums

Nutrition Facts
Serving Size 2 medium

Amount Per Serving

Calories 80	Calories from Fat 10

	% Daily Value*
Total Fat 1g	**1%**
Saturated Fat 0g	**0%**
Cholesterol 0mg	**0%**
Sodium 0mg	**0%**
Potassium 220mg	**6%**
Total Carbohydrate 19g	**6%**
Dietary Fiber 2g	**8%**
Sugars 21g	
Protein 1g	

Vitamin A 6%	•	Vitamin C 20%
Calcium 0%	•	Iron 0%

*Percent Daily Values are based on a 2,000 calorie diet. Your daily values may be higher or lower depending on your calorie needs.

**Contains less than 2% of the Daily Value of these nutrients.

Sweet Potatoes

Nutrition Facts
Serving Size 1 medium

Amount Per Serving

Calories 130	Calories from Fat 0

	% Daily Value*
Total Fat 0g	**0%**
Saturated Fat 0g	**0%**
Cholesterol 0mg	**0%**
Sodium 45mg	**2%**
Potassium 350mg	**10%**
Total Carbohydrate 33g	**11%**
Dietary Fiber 4g	**16%**
Sugars 7g	
Protein 2g	

Vitamin A 440%	•	Vitamin C 30%
Calcium 2%	•	Iron 2%

*Percent Daily Values are based on a 2,000 calorie diet. Your daily values may be higher or lower depending on your calorie needs.

**Contains less than 2% of the Daily Value of these nutrients.

Skim Milk

Nutrition Facts
Serving Size 1/2 pint (236 ml)
Servings Per Container 1

Amount Per Serving

Calories 90	Calories from Fat 0

	% Daily Value*
Total Fat 0g	**0%**
Saturated Fat 0g	**0%**
Cholesterol <5mg	**1%**
Sodium 130mg	**5%**
Total Carbohydrate 13g	**4%**
Dietary Fiber 0g	**0%**
Sugars 12g	
Protein 9g	

Vitamin A 10%	•	Vitamin C 2%
Calcium 30%	•	Iron 0%

*Percent Daily Values are based on a 2,000 calorie diet. Your daily values may be higher or lower depending on your calorie needs.

**Contains less than 2% of the Daily Value of these nutrients.

Chicken

Nutrition Facts
Serving Size 1 roasted drumstick
(61 g/about 2 oz.)
Servings Per Container 6

Amount Per Serving

Calories 110	Calories from Fat 50

	% Daily Value*
Total Fat 6g	**9%**
Saturated Fat 1.5g	**8%**
Cholesterol 85mg	**28%**
Sodium 50mg	**2%**
Total Carbohydrate 0g	**0%**
Protein 14g	**28%**
Iron	**4%**

Not a significant source of dietary Fiber, Sugars, Vitamin A, Vitamin C, or Calcium

*Percent Daily Values are based on a 2,000 calorie diet. Your daily values may be higher or lower depending on your calorie needs.

**Contains less than 2% of the Daily Value of these nutrients.

Reading the Food Label

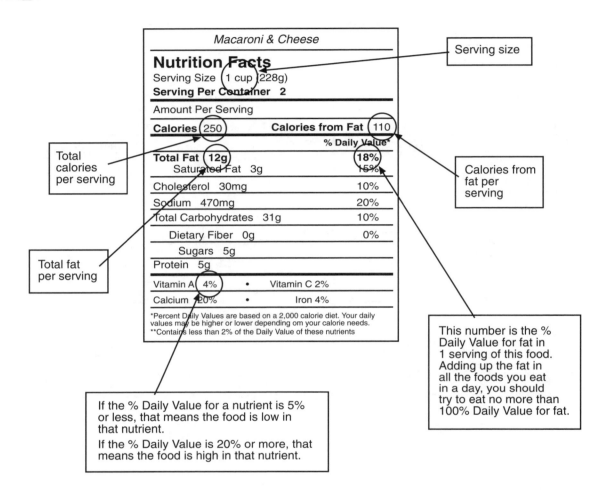

Serving size

Total calories per serving

Calories from fat per serving

Total fat per serving

Macaroni & Cheese

Nutrition Facts
Serving Size (1 cup (228g)
Serving Per Container 2

Amount Per Serving

Calories 250   **Calories from Fat** 110

% Daily Value*

Total Fat 12g	18%
Saturated Fat 3g	15%
Cholesterol 30mg	10%
Sodium 470mg	20%
Total Carbohydrates 31g	10%
Dietary Fiber 0g	0%
Sugars 5g	
Protein 5g	

Vitamin A 4%   •   Vitamin C 2%

Calcium 20%   •   Iron 4%

*Percent Daily Values are based on a 2,000 calorie diet. Your daily values may be higher or lower depending om your calorie needs.
**Contains less than 2% of the Daily Value of these nutrients

This number is the % Daily Value for fat in 1 serving of this food. Adding up the fat in all the foods you eat in a day, you should try to eat no more than 100% Daily Value for fat.

If the % Daily Value for a nutrient is 5% or less, that means the food is low in that nutrient.

If the % Daily Value is 20% or more, that means the food is high in that nutrient.

Can You Find It?

Name_____ Date_____

Nutrition Facts

Name of product _____

Serving size _____

Total fat per serving _____

% Daily Value of fat _____

% Daily Value of saturated fat _____

Nutrition Facts

Name of product _____

Serving size _____

Total fat per serving _____

% Daily Value of fat _____

% Daily Value of saturated fat _____

Nutrition Facts

Name of product _____

Serving size _____

Total fat per serving _____

% Daily Value of fat _____

% Daily Value of saturated fat _____

Nutrition Facts

Name of product _____

Serving size _____

Total fat per serving _____

% Daily Value of fat _____

% Daily Value of saturated fat _____

Nutrition Facts

Name of product _____

Serving size _____

Total fat per serving _____

% Daily Value of fat _____

% Daily Value of saturated fat _____

Nutrition Facts

Name of product _____

Serving size _____

Total fat per serving _____

% Daily Value of fat _____

% Daily Value of saturated fat _____

Nutrition Facts

Name of product _____

Serving size _____

Total fat per serving _____

% Daily Value of fat _____

% Daily Value of saturated fat _____

Nutrition Facts

Name of product _____

Serving size _____

Total fat per serving _____

% Daily Value of fat _____

% Daily Value of saturated fat _____

Snack Decisions

Background

There are no "bad" foods that should never be eaten; but most Americans eat too many foods high in saturated and *trans* fats, salt, and refined sugar. Snack foods tend to have a lot of saturated and *trans* fats, salt, and refined sugars. The reason the Food Guide Pyramid puts these types of foods at the top is because we already eat too much of these foods and not enough foods from the bottom of the pyramid—the fruits, vegetables, and whole grain groups.

The purpose of this lesson is to help students make better snack choices by recognizing sources of fat—especially sources of saturated fat (which is solid at room temperature) and *trans* fat (partially hydrogenated vegetable oils and shortenings and animal fats). It is important to remember that most saturated fats come from animal sources (including beef, chicken, pork, and dairy products). The few exceptions are coconut oil and palm oil, which are also rich in saturated fats. Since many baked or fried foods are prepared with partially hydrogenated vegetable oils, they also are sources of *trans* fat. Reading ingredient lists on food labels is an effective way to compare the fat and nutrient content of various snack foods.

The column on the food label headed "% Daily Value" can quickly tell you if a food is high or low in the nutrients listed. If the % Daily Value is 5 or less, the food is considered low in that nutrient. If the % DV is 20 or more, the food is high in that nutrient.

Whether or not the food fits into your diet depends on what other foods you eat. For most people, the daily goal is to choose foods that add up to about 100% of the Daily Value for total dietary fiber, vitamins, and minerals (especially vitamins A and C, calcium, and iron). For fat, saturated fat, cholesterol, and sodium, the goal should be to choose foods that add up to *no more than* 100% of the Daily Value. (To calculate %DV for fat, see lesson 5, page 60. The % Daily Value is based on a diet of 2,000 calories per day.)

The ingredients list on the food package lists ingredients in descending order of quantity (by weight). From this list, we can identify *trans* fat and added sugars. We can also get an idea of the quantity of these ingredients from their relative positions on the list. Ingredients such as vegetable shortening, partially hydrogenated soybean oil, and partially hydrogenated cottonseed oil are sources of *trans* fat. It is best to minimize the consumption of foods that contain *trans* fat. Added sugars come in many forms. Besides "sugar" (i.e., sucrose), high-fructose corn syrup and dextrose (glucose) are also examples of added sugar.

Estimated Teaching Time and Related Subject Area

Estimated teaching time: 1 hour, 10 minutes

Related subject area: language arts

Objectives

1. Students will examine a list of food selections to identify those with high nutritional value.
2. Students will be able to apply the "Collect-Consider-Compare-Decide" model when making decisions concerning choices of snack foods.
3. Students will create an advertisement or slogan for a healthy food choice.

Materials

1. Decision-making steps written on large poster board:

   Collect information.

   Consider nutrients.

   Compare for other choices.

   Make a decision.

2. Transparency #1, "Reading Food Labels"
3. Worksheet #1, "Healthy Snacks Vending Machine Company"
4. Handout #1, "Common Snacks Nutrient Chart"
5. Sample snack food labels

Procedure

Part I

1. Tell students that sometimes during work or school hours, people take a break. This break may be called a snack break, rest break, or time-out break.
2. Have students say what they think happens during a break from work or play. List students' suggestions on the board.
3. Have students tell why a pause or break is a healthy practice. (Emphasize that the body's needs—such as rest and food—may be addressed during breaks.)
4. Have students name some snacks they might enjoy during a work or play break. Write down students' choices on the board.

Part II

1. Tell students they will be in charge of choosing snacks for the machines from the "Healthy Snacks Vending Machine Company."

   Scenario: "The workers need snacks that will strengthen bones and muscles and give them lots of vitamins A, B, and C. Since workers need to be able to do a lot of lifting and have to work for long hours, they want snacks that will also give them energy."

2. Display the decision-making steps (on poster board).
3. Show the transparency "Reading Food Labels." Discuss % Daily Value with students and tell them that the % Daily Value is a good tool for helping them choose healthy snacks.

   The % Daily Value that appears on food labels lets them find out whether a food is high or low in a nutrient. Regarding total and saturated fat, if the % Daily Value is 5 or less for individual foods, then the food is considered low in that type of fat. The more foods chosen that have a % Daily Value of 5 or less for fats, the easier it is to eat a healthier diet. The overall daily goal (for all the foods they eat in a day) should be to select foods that together do not exceed 100% of the Daily Value for total and saturated fats.

   The % Daily Value also lets them find out whether a food is high or low in other nutrients, like vitamins A and C, calcium, and iron. If the %DV for any of these nutrients is 5 or less, it is considered low in that nutrient. If the % DV is 20 or higher, it is considered high in that nutrient. The overall daily goal (for all the foods they eat in a day) should be to select foods that together reach 100% of the Daily Value for these nutrients.

4. Select one of the suggested snacks from the students' list. Lead students in applying the following step-by-step process to determine if it is a healthy choice. (See nutrient chart, Handout #1.)

Decision-Making Process:

Collect information: Study the label or read nutrient chart (Handout #1).

Consider nutrients: Think about the nutrient content. Healthful snacks need to be (1) low in saturated and *trans* fats, (2) good sources of vitamins and minerals, (3) moderate to low in added sugar, and (4) moderate to low in salt.

Compare other choices: What other choices do I have? Is there a better selection?

Make a decision: What is best for the body? Is this selection low in saturated and *trans* fats? Is it from the broadest sections of the pyramid (grains, fruits, vegetables)?

5. Distribute the "Healthy Snacks Vending Machine Company" worksheet and "Common Snacks Nutrient Chart" and/or sample snack food labels. Have the students work in pairs or small groups to examine selections from the list of snacks available for the break. Ask the students to apply the decision-making process and come up with several healthy snacks for the vending machine. Students should be able to explain why they decided certain snacks were healthy and others were not.

6. After the pairs or groups have decided which snacks will be in their vending machines, have them share some of their findings with the rest of the class, referring to the steps of the model to explain their choices.

For example: "One of the snacks we analyzed was an orange. We consider this a good choice because we want something that is loaded with nutrients as well as calories. We found that an orange has a lot vitamin C, about 100% the Daily Value."

or

"We examined M&M candies as a snack. M&Ms have a lot of added sugar, so they gave some energy, but the energy probably didn't last long. Also, they have no vitamins or minerals, so they didn't give our bodies any healthy nutrients. We decided that M&Ms wouldn't be a healthy choice."

Summary

Have students write a persuasive letter or create an advertisement for one of the healthful snack choices they selected. The advertisement may be a poster (e.g., for a magazine or billboard) or a skit, rap, or song (for radio or television).

Extensions

1. Have students write a letter to the cafeteria manager requesting permission to display healthy snacks posters in the cafeteria.

2. Have students create a nutrition crossword puzzle that reinforces the important aspects of choosing healthful snacks. The puzzle may also contain nutrition and physical activity information learned in previous lessons.

3. Have students record the number of unhealthful snacks advertised on television during a given period. Also ask them to watch for the advertisements in other places, such as on billboards, on the radio, in magazines, etc.

4. Present two food labels to students (one a choice high in saturated fat—e.g., butter cookies—and one a low-fat choice—e.g., pretzels) and have students write a paragraph explaining why one is a better choice than the other for someone trying to eat a diet low in saturated fat.

5. Have students examine ingredient lists from food packages and identify sources of *trans* fat and added sugars.

1 Reading Food Labels

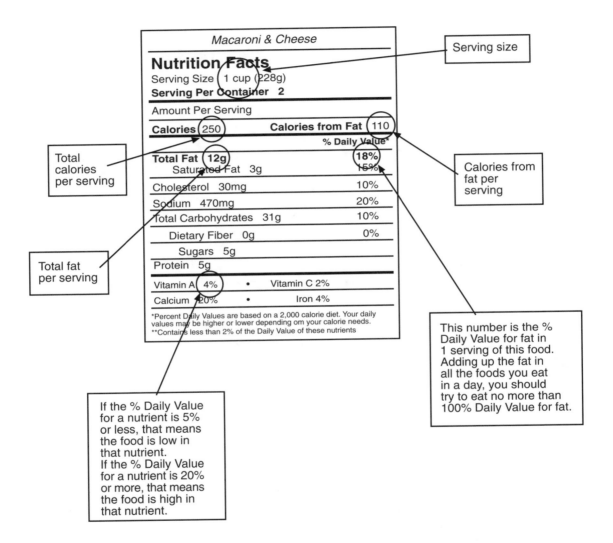

Serving size

Macaroni & Cheese

Nutrition Facts
Serving Size 1 cup (228g)
Serving Per Container 2

Amount Per Serving

Calories 250   **Calories from Fat** 110

% Daily Value*

Total Fat 12g   **18%**
    Saturated Fat 3g   15%

Cholesterol 30mg   10%

Sodium 470mg   20%

Total Carbohydrates 31g   10%

    Dietary Fiber 0g   0%

    Sugars 5g

Protein 5g

Vitamin A 4%   •   Vitamin C 2%

Calcium 20%   •   Iron 4%

*Percent Daily Values are based on a 2,000 calorie diet. Your daily values may be higher or lower depending om your calorie needs.
**Contains less than 2% of the Daily Value of these nutrients

Total calories per serving

Total fat per serving

Calories from fat per serving

This number is the % Daily Value for fat in 1 serving of this food. Adding up the fat in all the foods you eat in a day, you should try to eat no more than 100% Daily Value for fat.

If the % Daily Value for a nutrient is 5% or less, that means the food is low in that nutrient.
If the % Daily Value for a nutrient is 20% or more, that means the food is high in that nutrient.

Healthy Snacks Vending Machine Company

Directions

Write the names of your final snack choices in the spaces below.

Common Snacks

Table 17.1   Common Snacks

Snack	Total Calories	Added Sugar (g)	Fat (g)	Vit. A (IU)	Vit. C (mg)	Calcium (mg)	Iron (mg)	Sodium (mg)
		%Daily Value	%Daily Value	%Daily Value	%Daily Value	%Daily Value	%Daily Value	%Daily Value
Potato chips (1 oz. bag)	153	—	9.8	—	10	8	0.55	207
			15%	—	17%	1%	3%	9%
Cheese puffs (1 oz. bag)	159	—	10.0	83	1	17	0.75	368
			15%	2%	2%	17%	4%	15%
Hostess choc. cupcake (2)	314	59	8.8	2		43	1.37	490
			14%	0%		4%	8%	20%
Popcorn, unbuttered (1 cup)	54	—	0.7	—	.06	2	0.4	Trace
			1%	—	0%	0%	2%	—
Peanuts, salted (1 oz.)	170	—	14	Trace	Trace	10	—	138
			22%	—	—	1%	—	6%
Mixed nuts (8-12 nuts)	94	—	8.9	—	Trace	14	0.5	2
			14%	—	—	1%	3%	0%
Pear (1 medium)	98	—	.7	33	7	19	0.41	1
			1%	0%	12%	2%	2%	0%
Peanut butter cookies (2)	100	12	5.2	30	—	24	0.38	114
			8%	0%	—	2%	2%	5%
Cola (12 oz.)	159	369	—	—	—	—	—	—
			—	—	—	—	—	—

Snack	Added Total Calories	Sugar (g)	Fat (g)	Vit. A (IU)	Vit. C (mg)	Calcium (mg)	Iron (mg)	Sodium (mg)
		%Daily Value	%Daily Value	%Daily Value	%Daily Value	%Daily Value	%Daily Value	%Daily Value
Oatmeal cookies (2)	160	24	6.4	—	0.06	14	—	138
			10%	—	0%	1%	—	6%
Peppermint patties (1oz.)	124	25	2.3	—	—	—	—	—
			4%	—	—	—	—	—
M&M candies (1.5 oz.)	220	31	10	—	—	—	—	—
			15%	—	—	—	—	—
Chocolate chip cookies (2)	92	13	5.4	8	—	6	0.50	42
			8%	0%	—	1%	3%	2%
Sunflower seeds (1 oz.)	157	—	13.2	—	14	34	1.99	8
			20%	—	23%	3%	11%	0%
Orange (1 medium)	59	—	0.40	278	59	48	0.11	—
			0%	6%	98%	5%	1%	—
Orange juice, frozen (8 oz.)	112	—	0.10	194	97	22	0.24	2
			0%	4%	162%	2%	1%	0%
Carrots (1 large)	42	—	0.20	11,000	8	37	0.70	37
			0%	220%	13%	4%	4%	2%

(continued)

Table 17.1 *(continued)*

Snack	Total Calories	Added Sugar (g)	Fat (g)	Vit. A (IU)	Vit. C (mg)	Calcium (mg)	Iron (mg)	Sodium (mg)
		%Daily Value	%Daily Value	%Daily Value	%Daily Value	%Daily Value	%Daily Value	%Daily Value
Hot dog	273	—	15	—	11	75	1.5	868
			23%	—	18%	8%	8%	36%
Celery sticks (1 stalk)	8	—	0.01	120	5	20	0.20	63
			0%	2%	8%	2%	1%	3%
Pretzels (1.5 oz. bag)	166	—	1.5	—	—	10.5	0.80	676
			2%	—	—	1%	4%	28%
Doughnut (sugar icing) (1)	151	22	7	3	—	12	—	133
			11%	0%	—	1%	—	6%
Banana (1 medium)	105	—	0.6	92	10	7	0.35	1
			1%	2%	17%	1%	2%	0%
Apple (1 medium)	81	—	0.5	74	8	10	0.25	1
			0%	1%	13%	1%	1%	0%
Milk—1% (1 cup)	102	—	2.6	500	2	300	.12	122
			4%	10%	3%	30%	0%	5%
Grapes (1 cup)	58	—	0.3	92	4	13	0.27	2
			0%	2%	7%	1%	2%	0%
Hamburger (McDonald's)	255	—	9.8	82	2	51	2.3	520
			15%	2%	3%	5%	13%	22%

Snacking and Inactivity

Background

Students need energy to think, learn, and grow. Snacks are a very important part of a growing youth's diet. The usual snacks students choose, however, are not optimal for good health. Chips, soda, and other high-fat/high-sugar/high-salt foods are the items on which students most frequently snack. It is important that students choose snacks that are low in saturated and *trans* fats and high in the nutrients the body needs for good health (like fruits, vegetables, whole grains, low-fat dairy products, and 100% juices).

At the same time, students must also be encouraged to be physically active—to keep moving. More and more students spend their days in inactive ways. In an average year, students will spend more time watching TV than attending school.

It is therefore not only important for students to snack on nutritious foods—it is also important that they choose to be physically active more often. This is the topic of the following lesson: the importance of healthful snacking and physical activity.

This lesson stresses the importance of making healthy snack choices and the importance of being physically active. In the first part of the lesson, the teacher and class discuss the students' actual snacking and physical activity habits. In the second part of the lesson, students play the "Snack-n-Act" game, in which they are asked to pick out healthful snacks and activities from a pile of healthful and unhealthful choices. Before the game, students are guided through a warm-up exercise. After the game, students are guided through a cool-down session.

Estimated Teaching Time and Related Subject Areas

Estimated teaching time: 1 hour

Related subject areas: physical education, language arts

Objectives

1. The students will be able to choose a variety of healthy snacks.
2. The students will identify snacks that are less nutritious.
3. The students will identify active and inactive after-school pastimes.
4. The students will perform an endurance workout while pacing themselves during the fitness activity.
5. The students will demonstrate a pace that works for them so they can move for a long time without stopping.

Materials

1. Nutritious (low in saturated and *trans* fats, high in fiber) and less nutritious (high-fat or high-sugar) snack cards
2. Active after-school pastime and inactive after-school pastime cards
3. Ten boxes (places to put cards)—five with smiley faces, five with frowns
4. Diagrams of stretches (see appendix, pp. 453-456)

Procedure

1. Discuss the following with students: Do they snack after school? Why do they snack after school? What snacks do they eat?

2. Review the Food Guide Pyramid and snacks that come from the different food groups.

3. Discuss the following with students: What do they do after school? Do they have active lifestyles or inactive lifestyles?

4. If students are snacking for energy, what are they doing with the energy? Are they sitting around or are they using the extra energy?

5. Lead students in warm-up and stretching exercises.

   a. **Warm-up:** the first part of the safe workout, in which slow movements get the body ready for stretching and the fitness activity

      What to emphasize

      • Car analogy: your body is like a cold car—warm it up and then move it!

      • If you do not warm up, you are more likely to get injured.

      • You should always warm up before exercising, even when you are at home.

      • Always do the movements very slowly to warm up.

      • For example, for a bike ride, warm up by riding slowly at first.

      • Likewise, when throwing a ball, throw slowly at first.

   b. **Stretch:** The part of the safe workout in which you do exercises that improve flexibility fitness and get the body ready for the fitness activity (see diagrams in appendix, pp. 453-456)

      What to emphasize

      • Stretching improves flexibility fitness.

      • Activities such as riding a bike or doing push-ups do not improve flexibility.

      • Even if you aren't going to be doing a fitness activity, stretch at home while watching TV or when doing nothing in particular.

      • Hold stretches for 10 or more seconds.

      • Use slow movements; don't bounce.

6. Explain the "Snack-n-Act" game to students. The purpose of this game is to stress the importance of healthy snacking and of being physically active. We are also playing the game so that we can learn the importance of nonstop movement. Endurance fitness activities are very important for a healthy body.

7. Have the students form five groups and have them stand in lines. Place a variety of the nutritious snack cards, unhealthy snack cards, active after-school pastime cards, and the inactive after-school pastime cards on the opposite side of the room.

8. In front of each group line, place a box with a smiley face and one with a frown face. Tell the students about the food and activity cards located on the opposite side of the room.

9. Tell students that to play the game, each group member (one by one) will jog across the room, pick a food or activity card, jog back to the line, and place the card in the appropriate box. Each group has a box with a smiley face on it and a box with a frown—the frown box is for the unhealthy snack and inactive after-school pastime choices, while the smiley box is for the healthy snack and active after-school pastime choices.

10. Begin the game. Tell the students they should jog in place while waiting for their turn. Remember to stress that students should pace themselves.

11. Keep the game going until each group has received four or five turns (depending on how much time you have).

12. When the game is over, lead students in a cool-down session.

   a. **Cool-down:** The part of the safe workout in which your body slows down and recovers from the fitness activity.

   What to emphasize

   - Move slowly. Walking is an excellent cool-down activity.
   - Remember to cool down after exercising at home too.

   b. **Cool-down stretch:** The last part of the safe workout in which you do exercises that improve flexibility fitness (see the appendix).

   What to emphasize

   - Stretching after an activity is especially important; it improves flexibility fitness and helps you recover faster.
   - Activities such as riding a bike or doing push-ups do not improve flexibility.
   - Hold stretches for 10 or more seconds.
   - Use slow movements; don't bounce.

13. After the cool-down, review the contents of the boxes. Discuss any wrong choices.

Nutritious Snack Choices

apples

grapes

100%
fruit juice

frozen
fruit bars

low-fat
cheese

low-fat
crackers

cereal

English
muffins

melon	carrot sticks
whole wheat toast	cucumber slices
vegetable soup	low-fat yogurt
bagels	low-fat yogurt shake

low-salt pretzels	air-popped popcorn
banana	rice cakes
turkey sandwich	

Unhealthy Snack Choices

soda	potato chips
cookies	cake
candy	cheese doodles
brownies	cup cakes

pie	ice cream
fruit punch	candy bars
milk shakes	french fries
licorice	Pop Tarts

Active After-School Pastimes

bike riding	jumping rope
walking	running
skating	swimming
basketball	dancing

doing chores	playing catch
tossing a Frisbee	playing baseball
playing kickball	playing soccer
playing tag	playing hopscotch

Inactive After-School Pastimes

watching TV	sitting on the couch
playing video games	watching music videos
watching movies	sitting around doing nothing
lying on the couch	getting a ride everywhere

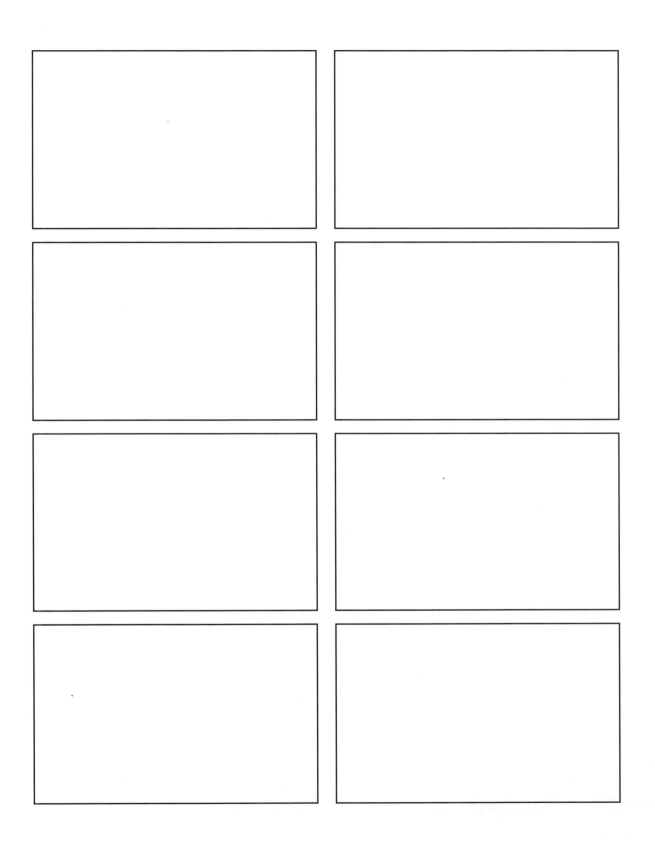

Freeze My TV

Background

During the late 1980s and early 1990s, 26% of all children watched over four hours of TV a day. For many children, watching TV has become a full-time job! On average, youth spend more time watching television each year than they spend in school.

This tendency toward an inactive or sedentary lifestyle is a contributing factor to youths' being overweight. On its own, television viewing is associated with elevated cholesterol levels and poor cardiovascular fitness in youth. Young people should be encouraged to consider healthy alternatives to television viewing, particularly those that involve more physical activity.

Estimated Teaching Time and Related Subject Areas

Estimated teaching time: 1 hour, 15 minutes

Related subject areas: math, language arts, art, social studies

Objectives

1. Students will analyze their leisure time to identify periods spent watching television.
2. Students will create a list of alternative activities to consider instead of television viewing.

Materials

1. Transparency #1, "Couch Potato"
2. Transparency #2, "Instead of Watching TV, I Could:"
3. TV guide/section of newspaper
4. Worksheet #1, "Television Blackout Tracking"
5. Colored stick-on dots (optional)

Procedure

Part I: Motivation

1. Display the transparency with the words "Couch Potato" on it, and ask students to discuss the message.
2. Have students suggest as many words or phrases as possible to describe a couch potato. You may want to use a web or other graphic organizer to record their suggestions.
3. Have students make comments regarding their television-viewing habits by identifying shows that they frequently watch.
4. Ask students if they think they can be called a "couch potato." Have them explain why or why not.

Part II: Concept Development

1. Display a television guide and have students brainstorm a list of their favorite weekday television programs. (Note: As list is compiled, help students add to the list by recalling programs that may have been left out.)

2. Record responses on a blackboard chart with columns for each of the seven days of the week. Be certain to list shows under the appropriate day of the week.

3. Have students review the list of programs and write down their three to five favorites for each day. Have them rate the shows, placing a number 1 next to their most favorite show and a number 5 next to their fifth favorite show, etc. (Note: This activity may be lengthy. It may be initiated in class but finished independently when students have completed other assigned work. Be certain that students have identified their three to five favorites for at least day 1 and day 2.)

4. After days 1 and 2 have been completed, have students circle the numbers indicating the two shows (one per day) they would have the least difficulty giving up. (These will probably be the shows they ranked as their fourth or fifth favorite.)

5. Conduct a brief discussion with students about why watching less TV and participating in more active alternatives might be beneficial to their health. (Encourage them to include the ideas that they are inactive and may tend to snack more while watching television than they might otherwise. Watching TV also provides less time to socialize with friends or family.)

Part III: Application

1. Display the "Instead of Watching TV, I Could:" transparency. Ask the students to brainstorm a list of alternative activities that they could do if they were not watching television. Encourage them to include all sorts of alternatives, such as hobbies, games, music, sports, reading, exercising, etc.

2. Write suggestions on the transparency. Have students indicate whether each suggested alternative involves physical activity (such as dancing, running, or playing basketball) or no physical activity (such as reading or playing a board game).

3. After students have evaluated and described each activity, discuss activities in terms of whether or not they are "heart-healthy" (provide exercise for the heart).

4. Have students estimate the number of hours in their day that could be classified as inactive. (Have a student discuss the meaning of the word.) Have students make bar graphs or pie charts to compare their inactive waking hours to the time during the day that they are active. These graphs or charts can be used to emphasize the need to increase physical activity.

Part IV: Television Blackout Tracking

1. Referring to their previous list of their top-ranked three to five shows for each day, have the students write the names of the shows on the Television Blackout Tracking sheet. Instruct students to circle the name of at least one show that they agree to give up each day.

2. Have the students review the "Instead of Watching TV, I Could:" list (above) and select those activities that they would like to try instead of watching television during one of their "blackout" times. Each will write the alternative activities in the "alternatives" spaces below the shows to be missed.

3. Tell students that they are asked to give up at least one 30-minute TV program each day. This is their TV "blackout" time. Explain that the following day each will

share with the rest of the students what he/she did as an alternative to watching TV.

4. Optional: A red sticker may be placed over the blackout selection on the tracking sheet if the student successfully gives up at least one 30-minute show per night. Give the students one sticker for each 30 minutes of TV they give up. Note: Students who are not successful should be encouraged to try again the next day.

Part V: Follow-Up

1. *Freeze My TV* promotion: Discuss promotion with students (see "Freeze My TV," lesson 25).

2. Have students create a poster illustrating their involvement in an alternative activity during a blackout period, encouraging others to try similar activities instead of watching television.

3. Have students write a letter to a friend discussing their self-selected alternatives to watching television and how changing television-watching habits could affect their lives.

4. Ask students to estimate the amount of time they have spent watching television in their lifetimes, including video games played on the television screen, and explain how they came up with their answer.

5. Have students interview older relatives or neighbors about what they did as children to entertain themselves. As a class or in small groups compile a "Catalog of Activities."

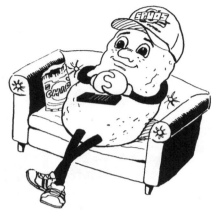

Couch
potato

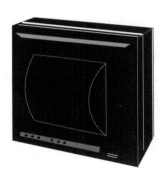

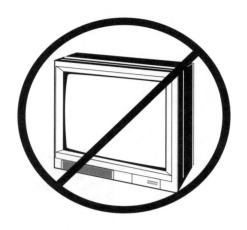

Instead of watching
television I could:

_____   _____

_____   _____

_____   _____

_____   _____

_____   _____

_____   _____

_____   _____

_____   _____

_____   _____

_____   _____

Television Blackout Tracking

Name _____

Directions

For each day, write in the television shows you usually watch. Circle one show each day to give up.

Table 19.1   Television Blackout Tracking Chart

Monday	Tuesday	Wednesday	Thursday	Friday	Saturday	Sunday

Alternatives

Menu Monitoring

Background

The GET 3-AT-SCHOOL & 5-A-DAY promotion, which encourages students to eat more fruits and vegetables, can be used as an extension to this lesson. See lesson 26 in part III, Promotions for the Classrom, for details.

Whole grain products, vegetables, and fruits are key parts of a varied and healthful diet. They provide vitamins, minerals, complex carbohydrates (starch and dietary fiber), and other substances that are important for good health. They are also generally low in saturated and *trans* fats, depending on how they are prepared and what is added to them at the table. Most Americans of all ages eat fewer than the recommended number of servings of grain products, vegetables, and fruits, even though consumption of these foods is associated with a substantially lower risk for many chronic diseases, including certain cancers, high blood pressure, and heart disease.

Most fruits and vegetables are naturally low in fat and provide many essential nutrients and other food components important for health. These foods are excellent sources of vitamin C, vitamin B_6, carotenoids (including those that form vitamin A), and folate. The antioxidant nutrients found in plant foods (e.g., vitamin C, carotenoids, vitamin E, and certain minerals) are of great interest to scientists and the public because of their potentially beneficial role in reducing the risk for cancer and certain other chronic diseases. Scientists are also trying to determine if other substances in plant foods protect against cancer, high blood pressure, and heart disease.

What Are the Main Benefits of Fruits and Vegetables?

- They are important sources of vitamins and minerals.
- They are important sources of fiber.
- They are low in saturated and *trans* fats.
- Research has shown that they reduce the risk of certain forms of cancer.

The availability of fresh fruits and vegetables varies by season and region of the country, but frozen and canned fruits and vegetables ensure a plentiful supply of these healthful foods throughout the year.

The 5-A-Day campaign promotes consumption of *at least* two servings of fruits and three servings of vegetables every day. The Food Guide Pyramid recommends two to three servings of fruits and three to four servings of vegetables every day. Fried potatoes (French fries and potato chips), because of their high fat content (especially saturated and *trans* fats), should not be counted toward the 5-A-Day goal.

Estimated Teaching Time and Related Subject Areas

Estimated teaching time: 50 minutes

Related subject areas: math, science, language arts, music

Objectives

1. Students design a day's menu of fruits and vegetables, making sure their menu choices include at least five selections of fruits and vegetables.
2. Students identify the nutritional values of certain fruits and vegetables.

Materials

1. Handout #1, "5 A Day"
2. Handout #2, "What They Do For Me (Vitamins and Minerals)"
3. Worksheet #1, "Plan a Menu & How Do You Rate?"
4. Worksheet #2, "Create a Frozen Food Item" (optional)
5. Transparency #1, "The Food Guide Pyramid"
6. Transparency #2, "Vegetables and Fruits"
7. Solutions to worksheet #1
8. Green and orange crayons/markers

Procedure

Part I

1. Guide students in singing or reciting the lyrics to the "5 A Day" tune found on handout #1. This song is the first track on the "Jammin' 5 A Day Songs" cassette available from Dole Foods (see p. 304 for ordering information).
2. Have students tell
   - the message contained in the song,
   - the names of fruits and vegetables mentioned, and
   - the names of citrus fruits not mentioned in the song.
3. As an alternative, students could create their own song/rap about fruits and vegetables.

Part II

1. Have the students form pairs. Distribute worksheet #1, "Plan a Menu," and explain to students that each pair will plan a healthful, full-day menu of fruits and vegetables.
2. Have students recall the 5-A-Day Fruits and Vegetables goal. Display transparency #1, "The Food Guide Pyramid," to the class. Review with students that the Food Guide Pyramid recommends at least five servings of fruits and vegetables a day (two to four of fruits, and three to five of vegetables). Explain that they will evaluate their menu to determine if they are reaching their 5-A-Day goal.
3. Ask students why fried potatoes, such as French fries and potato chips, do not count toward their 5-A-Day goal. (Answer: Because they contain high amounts of fat, especially saturated and *trans* fats.)
4. Display transparency #2, "Vegetables and Fruits," to the class. Encourage them to think of creative ways to include several servings in their menus.
5. Explain to students that some dishes are "mixed dishes"—dishes that contain fruits or vegetables along with other foods—such as stews, vegetable pizza, and chicken salad. The fruits and vegetables in mixed dishes can add up to a serving (or more). For example, the vegetables on two slices of vegetable pizza are likely to be equal to one serving of vegetables (1/2 cup).
6. Give the pairs 10 to 15 minutes to design their menus and record their selections on worksheet #1, "Plan a Menu." If desired, students could plan an entire week's menu on a separate sheet.

7. After 10-15 minutes, distribute handout #2, "What They Do for Me," which lists the benefits of some of the vitamins and minerals in fruits and vegetables (iron, calcium, vitamins A and C). Go over the chart with the class and discuss why we need these vitamins and minerals.

Part III

1. Have students score their selections by using the "How Do You Rate?" evaluation scale on the "Plan a Menu" worksheet.

2. Have students review and discuss their rating and decide whether they need to increase the number of fruits and vegetables in their menu. Have students set a goal for increasing (or maintaining if they already eat at least 5-A-Day) the number of fruits and vegetables they eat daily.

NOTE: Although some foods from other parts of the pyramid (other than the fruit and vegetable food groups) have been chosen for the menu, they should not receive any points. The objective of the exercise is to highlight and reward selections of fruits and vegetables.

Part IV

1. Distribute and review worksheet #2, "Create a Frozen Food Item."

2. Have students write their own songs or raps about fruits and vegetables.

5 A Day

5 A Day, eat 5 A Day
We all know that's the healthy way
Fruits and vegetables they're OK
A healthy way is 5 A Day

Spinach, cabbage, and cauliflower
Green peppers, corn, and peas
Choose your very own favorite vegetables
Any five you please

5 A Day, eat 5 A Day
We all know that's the healthy way
Fruits and vegetables they're OK
A healthy way is 5 A Day

Grapefruit, oranges, and nectarines
Bananas and honeydews
Fruits for a snack or a fun dessert
Will make you happy too

5 A Day, eat 5 A Day
We all know that's the healthy way
Fruits and vegetables they're OK
A healthy way is 5 A Day

When you go to the grocery store next time
Keep fruits and vegetables on your mind
Fresh or frozen, even canned will do
However they come, they're good for you

When your family sits down to eat
You can have some fun
Play the game of 5 A Day
Count them one by one

5 A Day, eat 5 A Day
We all know that's the healthy way
Fruits and vegetables they're OK
A healthy way is 5 A Day

What They Do for Me

Table 20.1 Vitamins & Minerals

What's the Nutrient?	Where Can I Get It?	What Does It Do for Me?
Vitamins		
Vitamin A	Carrots, sweet potatoes, greens, kale, spinach	• Helps me see at night • Gives me healthy skin
Vitamin C	Oranges, grapefruit, tangerines, cantaloupe, mango, papaya, strawberries, broccoli, bell peppers, tomatoes, potatoes (with skin)	• Keeps my skin and tissue healthy • Keeps my gums healthy
Minerals		
Calcium	Low-fat milk, low-fat cheese, yogurt, broccoli, greens, tofu (bean curd)	Gives me strong bones and teeth
Iron	Lean red meat, whole wheat bread, spinach, liver, lima beans	Allows blood to carry oxygen to all my body parts

Plan a Menu

Directions

Design a fruit and vegetable menu that would allow you to get your 5-A-Day. Be sure to write down fruits and vegetables you could eat for breakfast, lunch, and dinner.

Table 20.2 **Spotlight on Fruits & Vegetables**

	Breakfast	Lunch	Dinner
Day 1			

How do you rate?

Add up your points on the *Vita-Miner Meter*

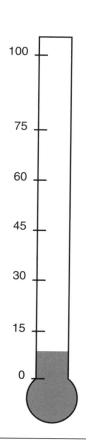

Vegetable	
_____	15 points
_____	15 points
_____	15 points
Total	_____

Fruit	
_____	15 points
_____	15 points
Total	_____

Total fruit	_____
Total vegetable	_____
Subtotal	_____
If subtotal is 75, add 25 bonus points	_____
Grand total	_____

Chart this on Vita-Miner Meter

Create a Frozen Food Item

You are the cook in charge of creating a new frozen food item. Your assignment is to make the new food item with ingredients that will help your body build strong bones, give you healthy skin, and help your body get the oxygen it needs. (Use the "What They Do for Me: Vitamins and Minerals" chart for guidance.)

1. Give your food product a name.
2. Write a short description of your new food product.
3. Write down the different types of foods you used (fruits, vegetables, and grains) and what each of these foods does for your body (for example, builds strong bones and healthy skin).
4. On the back page, design a container for your product.
5. Also on the back page, create a food label that includes the ingredients and nutrients in your food item.

New Product Name

_____

Description

_____

_____

_____

_____

_____

_____

_____

Food Guide Pyramid

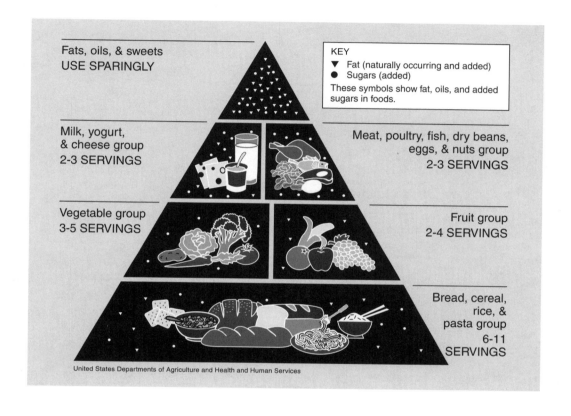

Vegetables and Fruits

Vegetables

Artichokes	Onions	
Asparagus	Okra	
Beans (string/lima)	Peas	
Beets	Potatoes	
Broccoli	Radishes	
Brussels sprouts	Rhubarb	
Cabbage	Seed sprouts	
Cauliflower	Spinach	
Carrots	Sweet corn	
Celery	Squash	
Cucumbers	Sweet potatoes	
Eggplant	Tomatoes	
Greens	Turnips	
Kale	Yams	
Leeks	Zucchini	
Lettuce		

Fruits

Apples

Apricots

Bananas

Blueberries

Cantaloupes

Cherries

Grapes

Grapefruits

Lemons

Mangoes

Nectarines

Oranges

Pears

Pineapples

Peaches

Raspberries

Strawberries

Tangerines

Watermelons

Solutions

Worksheet 1   Plan a Menu

Table 20.3   **Spotlight on Fruits and Vegetables Example**

	Breakfast	Lunch	Dinner
Day 1	Orange	Carrots Banana	Spinach Baked potato

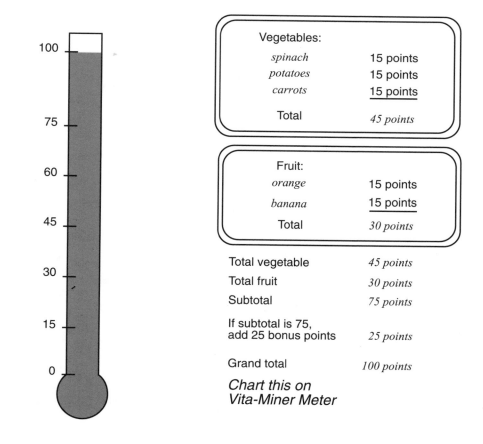

Vegetables:

spinach	15 points
potatoes	15 points
carrots	15 points
Total	*45 points*

Fruit:

orange	15 points
banana	15 points
Total	*30 points*

Total vegetable	*45 points*
Total fruit	*30 points*
Subtotal	*75 points*
If subtotal is 75, add 25 bonus points	*25 points*
Grand total	*100 points*

Chart this on
Vita-Miner Meter

The Game of Veggiemania

Background*

The four most popular vegetables in the United States are potatoes, tomatoes, iceberg lettuce, and onions. These vegetables, unfortunately, often end up as French fries, onion rings, or potato chips and as ketchup, lettuce, and onions on fast-food hamburgers.

While there is no such thing as a bad vegetable, some vegetables are more "nutrient-dense" than others, meaning they contain more nutrients, such as vitamins and minerals. The question, then, is which vegetables are more nutrient-dense than others. All vegetables are good, but in this lesson, students will be learning about which vegetables are very nutrient-dense.

Components that can be used to rate the nutrient density of vegetables include vitamins like vitamin C and folate, minerals (like potassium, calcium, iron), carotenoids (which act as antioxidants and can help reduce the risk of some forms of cancer), and fiber (which also can reduce the risk of some forms of cancer).

- **The top vegetables** (very nutrient-dense vegetables): broccoli, cabbage, carrots, chard, collard greens, green beans, kale, spinach, tomatoes
- **Good vegetables** (all the rest): asparagus, avocado, cauliflower, celery, corn on the cob, romaine lettuce, parsley, potatoes (baked), squash, sweet potatoes, alfalfa sprouts, beets, corn (frozen), eggplant, mushrooms, onions, radishes, turnips

The basic message is that all vegetables are good to eat, but some are better than others in terms of the nutrients and benefits they provide the body. Of the four most popular vegetables in the U.S. (potatoes, tomatoes, iceberg lettuce, and onions), only tomatoes could be categorized as "tops." Students (as well as everyone else) should be encouraged to eat more vegetables from the "tops" category.

* Partial source of background material: Center for Science in the Public Interest

Estimated Teaching Time and Related Subject Areas

Estimated teaching time: 60 minutes

Related subject areas: math, science

Objectives

1. The students will understand that all vegetables are good but that some are more nutrient-dense (and therefore more nutritious) than others.
2. Students will be able to distinguish those vegetables that are very nutrient-dense.
3. The students will demonstrate the parts of a safe workout while learning about nutrient density.

Materials

1. Five containers (such as bags or boxes)
2. Veggiemania cards (cards displaying names of vegetables)

   (Two copies of each card should be made so that there will be 50-60 cards that can be spread out, face up, on the opposite end of the room.)
3. Worksheet #1, "Let's Get to the Points"

Procedures

Part I

1. Ask the students to raise their hands if they have ever eaten any of the following vegetables:

Kale	Tomatoes
Spinach	Green beans
Carrots	Collard greens
Chard	Brussels sprouts
Eggplant	Squash
Broccoli	Cabbage

2. Explain to students that if they have eaten any of those vegetables, they have eaten some of the "best," the most healthy, and the most nutrient-dense vegetables they can for their bodies.

3. Explain to students that a nutrient-dense vegetable contains a lot of the vitamins and minerals our bodies need to grow, to be healthy, and to work right.

4. Discuss additional benefits of eating vegetables that are nutrient-dense. Such vegetables contain a lot of nutrients, especially vitamins A and C and fiber, which can help protect the body against cancer and heart diseases.

Part II

As in previous lessons, this lesson should follow the format of the safe workout.

1. Lead students through a warm-up and stretch.

   Warm-up: the first part of the safe workout in which slow movements get the body ready for stretching and the fitness activity

   Stretch: the part of the safe workout in which you do exercises that improve flexibility fitness and get the body ready for a fitness activity

2. Explain to students that they are going to participate in a fitness activity focusing on nutrient-dense vegetables.

   Fitness activity: the part of the safe workout in which strength and endurance fitness exercises are performed

3. Have the students form five groups.

4. Each group will be moving nonstop in a line, one behind the other. On one side of the classroom there should be five lines moving nonstop (pacing). Remind the students that eating right is only half the story, they must also be active!

5. Place a container next to each line into which the students will put their Veggiemania cards. (This and the next step can be done beforehand.)

6. On the opposite side of the classroom, spread out the Veggiemania cards on the floor, with the vegetable name facing up. (See line diagram, figure 21.1.)

7. Explain to the students that when you say "Go," the first person in each line should jog/walk to the other side of the room, and choose a Veggiemania card naming the most nutrient-dense vegetable he/she can find (without taking too much time), return (jogging/walking) to the line, put the card into the container, then go to the end of the line, where he/she should continue pacing (marching or jogging in place). The next student in line should take a turn as soon as the card is put in the bag.

Line diagram for lesson 21

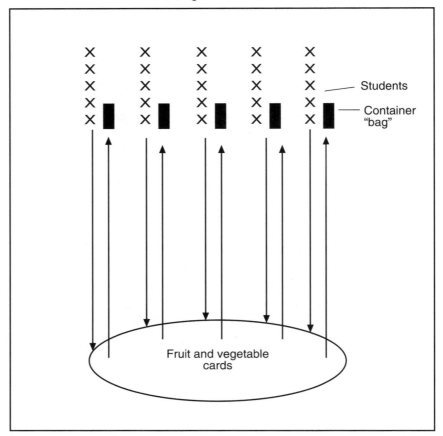

Figure 21.1   Line diagram for Lesson 21.

8. Teacher concludes the game once all of the cards have been picked up or when time is up (length of time is up to the teacher).

9. Lead students in a cool-down and cool-down stretch.

Cool-down: the part of the safe workout in which your body slows down and recovers from the fitness activity

Cool-down stretch: the last part of the safe workout in which you do exercises that improve flexibility fitness

10. Have each group sit around their container and remove the Veggiemania cards.

11. Distribute "Let's Get to the Points" worksheet to each group. Explain the vegetable point system to students and have each group add up the points on their cards and share their answers with the other groups.

12. Have each group share their 100-point ("Tops") cards and write these on the board. Encourage students to eat more of these types of nutrient-dense vegetables when they get their 5-A-Day of fruits and vegetables.

Let's Get to the Points

Date _____

Group Members _____

_____

Directions

Using the point system below, determine the points for each of your vegetable cards. Then add up the total points for all the cards.

Table 21.1   Veggiemania Card Points

	100-POINT CARDS
The Top Vegetables (very nutrient dense)	broccoli, cabbage, carrots, chard, collard greens, green beans, kale, spinach, tomatoes

	50-POINT CARDS
Good Vegetables (all the rest)	asparagus, avocado, celery, cauliflower, corn on the cob, romaine lettuce, parsley, potatoes (baked), sweet potatoes, squash, alfalfa sprouts, beets, corn (frozen), cucumbers, eggplant, iceberg lettuce, mushrooms, onions, radishes, turnips

Table 21.2   Veggiemania Score Card

Vegetable	Points		Vegetable	Points

Total Points for all Vegetables_____

Vegetable Cards

Tops

spinach	kale
collard greens	tomatoes
carrots	green beans
broccoli	cabbage
Swiss chard	

Good Vegetables (all the rest)

asparagus	avocado
cauliflower	celery
corn (fresh)	parsley
potato (baked)	romaine lettuce
squash	sweet potatoes

alfalfa sprouts	beets
corn (frozen)	eggplant
mushrooms	onions
radishes	turnips

Breakfast Bonanza*

Background**

Breakfast is the most important meal of the day. Eating breakfast gives the body the energy it needs to start the day and perform the morning's important tasks, from thinking to doing the dishes to working out. Generally, adults who eat breakfast regularly learned this lifelong good habit when they were children.

National studies show that children who eat breakfast are better prepared for the school day. They perform better in school, are tardy less often, and miss fewer days of school. Students who eat breakfast have also demonstrated that their ability to concentrate is better, their reaction times are faster, their energy levels are higher, and their scores on tests are better.

To help make breakfast a lifelong habit, students (and adults) should be encouraged to start their day by eating breakfast. Any good, nutritious food can be eaten for breakfast. If people don't happen to like typical breakfast foods, such as cereal or toast, they can eat leftovers from dinner, like pizza or a sandwich. The most important thing is to eat a nutritious meal in the morning.

Ideally, breakfast should contain a substantial amount of complex carbohydrates (from foods like whole grain cereal, toast, fruit, and 100% fruit juice) and some protein (preferably from nuts or low-fat dairy products like 1% milk or low-fat yogurt). This means eating from the bottom three layers of the Food Guide Pyramid—the grain group, fruits and vegetables groups, and low-fat dairy and protein groups.

The carbohydrates in a nutritious breakfast give the body energy, and the protein helps stave off a midmorning drop in blood sugar level that can make children lethargic before lunchtime. In a healthy person, blood sugar levels indicate how much fuel (in the form of glucose) is immediately available to the body. When blood sugar levels drop, children (and adults) may feel hungry, drowsy, and less energetic as well as have trouble concentrating. Breakfast can help keep blood sugar levels at the right level throughout the morning until lunchtime.

Foods such as doughnuts, colas, candy bars, and desserts contain a lot of simple sugars and are not the best choices for breakfast, because they can cause blood sugar levels to drop faster than foods containing complex carbohydrates and protein.

* Lesson adapted from Texas Education Agency Nutrition Education Curriculum Guide, Grade 5-8, and a lesson plan developed by Ms. Michele Dorsey.
** Partial source of background material: Maryland Food Committee.

Estimated Teaching Time and Related Subject Areas

Estimated teaching time: 1 hour

Related subject areas: math, science

Objectives

1. Students will able to discuss the importance of breakfast.
2. Students will be able to name nutritious breakfast foods.
3. Students will demonstrate their ability to calculate the measurements of an orange and to calculate the average of their findings.

Materials

1. Blank sheets of drawing paper or chart paper
2. Pencils, crayons, and/or colored markers
3. Rulers
4. Twine
5. Scale(s)
6. Graphic organizer
7. Calculators
8. Oranges (12)
9. Worksheet #1, "Measure Up!"
10. Passages: "Oranges," and "Have You Ever Heard of ...?"

Procedure

Part I: Language Arts Discussion (Importance of Breakfast)

1. Ask students why they think it is important to eat a nutritious breakfast. Write their responses on the board.

   Below are some examples of what studies have shown about breakfast:
   - People who skip breakfast do not perform as well in tasks of concentration as those who eat breakfast.
   - People who skip breakfast have shorter attention spans.
   - People who skip breakfast may feel drowsy by midmorning.
   - People who skip breakfast score lower on tests than those who eat breakfast.
   - People who skip breakfast are less energetic.

2. Explain to students that the body needs fuel in order to perform well. (You could have the fastest car in the world, but if it doesn't have any gas [fuel] it won't go anywhere.)

3. Discuss with students that the word breakfast means "breaking the fast." A "fast" is a long period without eating. After dinner and sleeping overnight, the body has gone 10 to 12 hours without food. By eating breakfast, you are breaking the overnight fast and giving your body the fuel (food) it needs to play, think, and have fun.

   If appropriate, remind students that breakfast is available to them before school in the cafeteria.

4. Ask students to name foods they enjoy eating for breakfast. Tell them that any nutritious foods may be eaten for breakfast—they don't have to eat only "breakfast foods." For example, leftover vegetable pizza, a turkey sandwich, rice and beans, and casseroles are all foods they can eat for breakfast.

5. Give each student a blank piece of paper. Instruct the students to write the letters of their name vertically. Next to each letter in their name, tell students to write the name of a food beginning with that letter.

   Suggest that they write down foods that they enjoy eating for breakfast.

   Example:

   Dates

   Apples

   Raisins

   Yogurt

   Loganberries

6. Pick a select number of students to share their answers. Ask some students who have an "O" in their names to share their answers. Did any of them come up with an "orange" for the "O?" Oranges and 100% orange juice are a good part of a nutritious breakfast.

7. Have students read aloud (in unison) the two short passages "Oranges for Each Day's Journey" and "Have You Ever Heard of …?" (both on page 256).

   Discussion questions relating to the passages:

   - Why do you think the author wrote the passage?
   - What is the main idea of the passage?
   - Name the places in the world where oranges grow.
   - What is meant by the term "Valencia"?
   - How did the blood orange get its name?
   - Why is it important to have vitamin C in your body?
   - How does vitamin C protect you?

Part II: Math Activity (Examining an Orange)

Note: For part II, the class must be able to use oranges. If oranges (or similar fruit) are unavailable, part II can be postponed until they are available.

1. Tell students that, now that they know why oranges are good for them nutritionally, they are going to learn even more about oranges by examining them scientifically.

2. Demonstrate to students how the circumference is the distance around the orange.

3. Show students that by placing a piece of string around the orange and then measuring the string, they will get an approximation of the circumference of the orange.

Additional Information

Explain the math formulas that can be used to determine the circumference of a circle.

Circumference = diameter $\times$ π

   or

Circumference = $2\pi r$

(π = 3.1416; r = radius)

4. Distribute worksheet #1 and have students work cooperatively to complete the questions, chart, and graph. (Their goal is to gather data and present their findings in an organized chart and graph.)

   Note: To help students approximate the weight of the orange, it may be helpful to mention how much other similar-sized items weigh (such as an apple or tennis ball).

5. Student will share in their journals what they learned about breakfast and oranges.

Measure Up!

Name_____ Date_____

Group members _____

_____

Table 22.1   The Orange

	Estimate	Your Measurements	Average of Group Members' Measurements
Weight (ounces)			
Sections (number)			
Seeds (number)			
Circumference (inches)			

Step 1

Answer these questions:

- How much do you think an average orange weighs? _____

- How many sections do you think are in an average orange? _____

- How many seeds do you think are in an average orange? _____

- What do you think is the circumference of an average orange? _____

Step 2

Write the answers from step 1 in the chart above in the "Estimate" column.

Step 3

a. Examine an actual orange to determine its weight, circumference, and number of seeds and sections. Write these findings in the "Your measurements" column.

b. Now average the findings of your group (hint: use calculators). Put these answers in the "Average of group members' measurements" column.

Step 4

In the examples on the next page, make bar graphs to display the estimates and actual answers. Use the chart paper and markers.

Attributes of an orange

Weight (ounces)

Number of sections

Number of seeds

Circumference

☐ Estimated   ■ Actual measurement

Passages

Oranges For Each Day's Journey

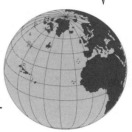

Oranges originally grew in Asia and the East Indies (do you know where these are on the map?), and were brought to Europe by explorers and then to the New World (North America).

The vitamin C in oranges and other citrus fruit (like lemons, limes, and grapefruit) helped to keep these early explorers, like Columbus, Magellan, and Marco Polo, healthy on their very long journeys across the seas. Just like the explorers, you can keep healthy and strong on your daily journeys (to school, home, and the store) by eating oranges and other citrus. It's as easy as pouring a glass of 100% juice or eating the orange wedges served in the cafeteria. You'll be energized to play, and the vitamin C will help you grow strong, heal cuts and bruises, and fight off infections.

Have You Ever Heard of Pineapple Oranges? How About Valencia, Temple, Navel, or Blood Oranges?

The oranges you usually see in the cafeteria are called pineapple oranges. These are popular because they have few seeds and have the familiar bright orange skin.

All types of oranges are sweet and juicy, but each has a different name and looks a little bit different from one another. Some are light orange on the inside, some are bright orange on the inside, and some are even bright red (these are called blood oranges).

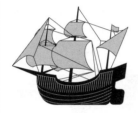

Some have thin skin and some have thick skin. They also come in different sizes, ranging from the smaller temple to the larger navel.

Because oranges are so delicious, they make a great snack—even a sweet dessert! You can eat them peeled or cut into wedges, like in the cafeteria, or you can "drink" them as 100% juice. Any of these ways lets you enjoy oranges and gives you a boost of vitamin C that helps you grow, play, and learn.

Foods From Around the World: Italy, China, Mexico, and Ethiopia

Background

Although all people of the world eat food because it provides them with nutrients and energy, they get their nutrients from many different types of foods prepared in many different ways. In the countries of Italy, Mexico, China, and Ethiopia, the types of food and patterns of eating are very different from those in the United States. Yet the traditional diets of each country can provide the nutrients people need to grow and stay healthy.

In Italy, the midday meal is the largest of the day and consists of several courses including an appetizer course called antipasto. Evening meals are traditionally light. Pizza was first served in Naples, a city in southern Italy, as a bread topped with tomatoes and mozzarella cheese. It is eaten as a light evening meal or as a snack. The Italians have not only given us pizza, but pastas and delicious cheeses.

Traditional foods in Mexico include corn tortillas, tomatoes, beans, rice, chocolate, and cheese. Canned and powdered milk is common. Traditionally, Mexicans eat breakfast, a main midday meal, and a light evening meal or snack. Tortillas are generally served at every meal as bread.

In China, rice is usually eaten with every meal, especially in southern China. Many cooks prepare it each morning and keep it on the stove ready to eat all through the day. Along with rice, many meals include seafood, chicken, soybean products, noodles, and vegetables.

People in Ethiopia typically eat one main meal in the evening. Lentils, other beans, teff (a kind of grain), bread, potatoes, fruit, and vegetables are a big part of their diets.

Experimenting with dishes from other countries can bring excitement to a meal as well as provide a whole new range of foods that can fit into a healthful diet and the recommendations of the Food Guide Pyramid.

Estimated Teaching Time and Related Subject Areas

Estimated teaching time: 60 minutes

Related subject areas: social studies, geography

Objectives

1. Students will understand that different foods are eaten in different countries around the world.
2. Students will be able to identify food choices from the countries of Mexico, China, Italy, and Ethiopia.
3. Students will discuss the different foods that would be found on the Food Guide Pyramid for each country.
4. Students will perform a safe workout while learning about multiethnic foods.

Materials

1. Maps of Mexico, China, Italy, and Ethiopia (provided)
2. Cards listing foods from each country (duplicate four sets of cards)
3. Four bags to hold the food cards

Procedure

As in previous lessons, this lesson should follow the format of the safe workout.

1. Lead students through a warm-up and stretch.

   Warm-up: the first part of the safe workout, in which slow movements get the body ready for stretching and the fitness activity

   Stretch: the part of the safe workout, in which you do exercises that improve flexibility fitness and get the body ready for a fitness activity

2. Explain to students that they are going to participate in a fitness activity focusing on foods from Italy, Mexico, China, and Ethiopia.

   Fitness activity: the part of the safe workout in which strength and endurance fitness exercises are performed

3. Have the class form four groups.

4. The students will be moving nonstop with their group in a line in the center of the room.

5. On the floor in each corner of the room, place one of the four maps. (This can be done beforehand.) Tell students which map has been placed in which corner and/ or hang a sign in the corner above each map.

6. Place a bag of food cards in front of each group. (For a summary of the food cards and the food groups to which they belong, see table 23.1, "Food Guide Pyramid Groups.")

7. Tell the students that on your signal, the first person in each line should take a food card out of his or her bag, walk/jog carefully to the map of the country from which that food comes, and place the card on it.

8. All students should continue to move in place nonstop until all of the food cards have been distributed about the room. Remind students to continue to move nonstop throughout the entire fitness activity.

9. After all the food cards have been placed on the maps, assign a country to each of the four groups.

10. Have each group go to their map and lead them in a cool-down and cool-down stretch.

    Cool-down: the part of the safe workout in which your body slows down and recovers from the fitness activity

    Cool-down stretch: the last part of the safe workout in which you do exercises that improve flexibility fitness

11. Have each group review the foods placed on their map to make sure all the foods belong there. If a group has questions about the placement of a food, they can ask you individually, or discuss it with the entire class during step #12.

12. Move to each map in the room and discuss the foods of each country and the Food Guide Pyramid groups to which they belong. Discuss combination foods (when a food contains more than one food group).

13. Using the food cards, discuss how the eating habits and choices of people in these other countries are different from or similar to the eating habits and food choices of people in the United States.

Table 23.1 Food Guide Pyramid Groups

Italian Food Cards

Food	Group	Food	Group
bread	grain	pasta primavera (pasta with veg.)	grain, veg., & fats
corn meal	grain	polenta (cornmeal)	grain
foccacia (flat bread)	grain	risotto (rice)	grain
fruits	fruit	vegetables	vegetable
olive oil	fats		

Chinese Food Cards

Food	Group	Food	Group
bean sprouts	vegetable	fresh fruit	fruit
chicken (roasted, baked, steamed)	meat	mi fan (rice noodles)	grain
chow mein (noodles)	grain	sautéed vegetables	veg. & fats
chow fan (noodles)	grain	tofu (bean curd)	meat
congee (rice pudding)	grain	Chinese cabbage	vegetable
fish	meat	won ton & bao (dumplings)	grain

Mexican Food Cards

Food	Group	Food	Group
beans	meat	corn	vegetable
beans and rice	meat & grain	pork	meat
beef	meat	rice	grain
beef burritos	meat & grain	tortillas (beans, meat & cheese)	grain, meat, & dairy
cheese	dairy	tostadas	grain
chicken enchiladas	meat & grain		

Ethiopian Food Cards

Food	Group	Food	Group
beans	meat	misir wat (lentil stew)	meat
bread	grain	potatoes	vegetable
fruits	fruit	shero wat (pea stew)	vegetable
lentils	meat	teff (a grain)	grain
gomen (collard greens)	vegetable	vegetables	vegetable

Food Cards

bread	pasta primavera (pasta with vegetables)
corn meal	polenta (cornmeal)
foccacia (flat bread)	risotto (rice)
fruits	vegetables
olive oil	

bean sprouts	fresh fruit
chicken (roasted, baked, steamed)	**mi fan** (rice noodles)
chow mein (noodles)	**sautéed vegetables**
chow fan (noodles)	**tofu** (bean curd)
congee (rice pudding)	**Chinese cabbage**

fish	won ton and bow (dumplings)
beans	corn
beans and rice	pork
beef	rice
beef burritos	tortillas (beans, meat, and cheese)

cheese	tostadas
chicken enchiladas	misar wat (lentil stew)
beans	potatoes
bread	

fruits	shero wat (pea stew)
lentils	teff (a grain)
gomen (collard greens)	vegetables

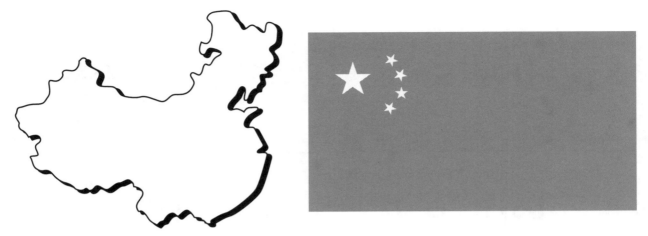

Figure 23.2a-b China and its flag.

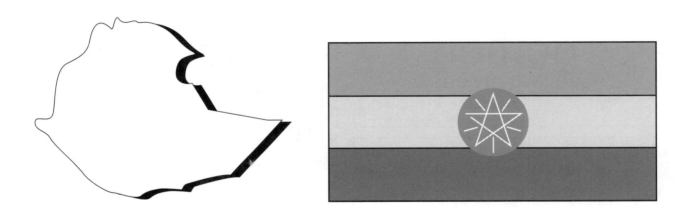

Figure 23.3a-b Ethiopia and its flag.

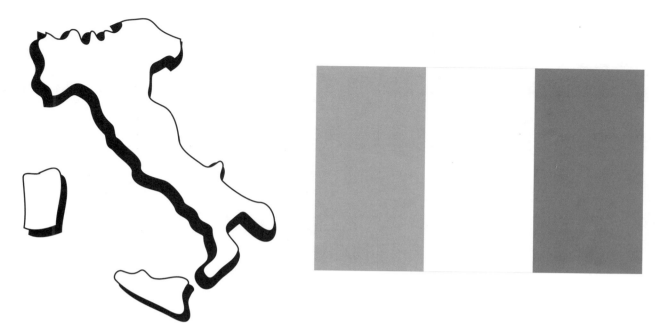

Figure 23.4a-b Italy and its flag.

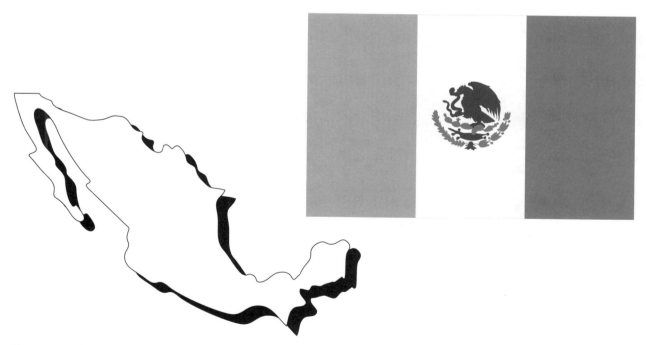

Figure 23.5a-b Mexico and its flag.

Fitness Walking

Background

Note: This lesson is a duplicate of lesson 12 in the grade 4 lesson-set. While the walking program aspect will be the same for both grades, the grade 4 and grade 5 lessons can be kept distinct by choosing a different social studies theme around which to plan the walking program.

Walking is one of the healthiest, safest, and easiest ways to begin a fitness program and can be a big step toward improving your health. Fitness or aerobic walking uses all of the major muscle groups in the upper and lower body in a nonimpacting, dynamic, rhythmic action, which is what an ideal exercise should do.

Walking is also free! There are no machines or membership fees, no fancy packaging or expensive clothes. Walking requires only that you "race" yourself and do your "personal best." What's important is feeling good about yourself and setting your own standards and goals.

Walking can be done with friends or family. It can also be done as an adventure with a school class. An active lifestyle can make you feel better, give you more energy, and enhance your health. We want you and your class to get hooked on walking. It's fun, and it's good for you!

Overview

This lesson introduces students to the benefits and fun of walking for fitness. The lesson also serves as a kickoff for an ongoing class-walking club that can be integrated into geography activities throughout the year.

Estimated Teaching Time and Related Subject Areas

Estimated teaching time: 1 hour

Related subject areas: science, social studies, math, physical education

Objectives

1. Students will learn about the importance of regular exercise and establish an ongoing class-walking club.
2. Students will be exposed to the benefits of walking with family, friends, and classmates.
3. Students will learn walking techniques and learn about the health benefits of raising one's heart rate through regular aerobic activity.
4. Students will learn about a particular geographic region of the world.

Materials

1. Comfortable shoes (students and teacher)
2. Worksheet #1, "Teacher Classroom Walking Log"
3. Worksheet #2, "Student Classroom Walking Log" (duplicate for students)
4. Worksheet #3, "Student Home Walking Log" (duplicate for students)
5. Map(s)
6. Map pins/thumb tacks

Preparation

Planning a Walking Club

In addition to introducing students to how important and fun walking can be, this lesson also focuses on the organization of a class-walking club.

When planning a walking club, first consider where and when your students can walk. The walks can take place before, during, or after school, and can be done in the hallways, gym, playgrounds, or around the neighborhood—whenever and wherever such a program works best for your school.

An effective way to introduce a walking club into your school would be to integrate it with your curriculum. One option is to integrate the club with your social studies curriculum—e.g., with lessons on the state in which you live, the entire United States, or other countries around the world. If there is an area of the world your students would like to learn about, use the walking club to help you accomplish this. As a class or individually, design the itinerary of a fitness walk across the region you have chosen to cover. Students could walk across America together, walk across a region of the U.S., or walk around the world. The design is completely open.

Give your program a name, such as "Walk Across America" or "Walk Across the World," or let the students choose a name or country.

Using maps of the area(s) you choose, tie in the students' walking progress with movement on the map. Each time the class walks a certain period of time, equate that with a particular distance on the map (for example, five minutes walked could equal 50 miles). Each student can have a map, or all of the students can plot their travels on one map. The amount of time the class walks and the distance traveled will depend on the part of the world or country on which you chose to focus. For example, if you decide on a large area of the world, such as Africa, then five minutes might equal 200 miles traveled. If you chose the state of Maryland, five minutes might equal 50 miles.

Keep track of your class walks on the logs provided. There is a log for each class, as well as for each student. The class log can be made larger and displayed in the classroom for all to see. Along with the log, display a map of the area/region/country across which they will be traveling. Displaying the map and log will motivate the class and keep everyone more involved.

Encourage students to take on the walking program as an after-school, family-and-friend adventure. Have the students keep a log of the dates and times of their after-school walks (see "Student Home Walking Log"). They can plot their travels on the maps with pins or thumb tacks. Get the whole school involved in walking—principals, office staff, custodians, and other teachers and students can become involved. The more the students see others participating, the more they will want to become involved.

Procedure

1. What Is Fitness Walking?

Explain to students that "fitness walking" is walking at a pace (speed) that makes the heart, lungs, and blood vessels work harder than usual. This type of aerobic workout makes the heart muscle pump harder because the body's other muscles—leg and arm muscles—are working harder and need more blood to keep them going.

Blood gives muscles energy to work. When muscles work hard, such as when you're doing fitness walking, they need more energy. During exercise, the heart works harder to pump blood to these muscles. When the heart works hard, it gets stronger.

Explain to students that they can check their pulse rate before they begin exercising and again during their fitness workout, in order to see firsthand how the heart muscle works harder. (See details on how to do this in the section "Finding a Pulse".)

2. Benefits of Fitness Walking

Ask students to list the benefits of fitness walking. These can include the following:

a. Walking is an excellent and safe way to achieve aerobic conditioning. Aerobic conditioning means taking care of the heart, lungs, and blood vessels. Walking lets you do this with less wear and tear on the body compared to many other types of conditioning.

b. Walking, like other aerobic exercises, can give you more energy and reduce fatigue.

c. Walking can help relieve stress.

d. Walking can improve mood and mental function.

e. Walking can help in weight control.

f. Walking can help slow down the progression of osteoporosis (bone loss), which can occur when one ages.

g. Walking can be performed with friends and family.

3. How to Fitness Walk

a. Make sure students wear sneakers or comfortable shoes.

b. Review with students the following:

1. **Arm swing:** Try to keep the arms swinging at a pace faster than they swing when walking normally. The faster the arms swing, the faster the legs will move. Bend the arms 90 degrees at the elbow. Concentrate on moving the arms faster and swinging them from the shoulder. Remember, when you shorten your arms (bending them at the elbow 90 degrees), you can swing them faster and your legs will move faster. Keep your shoulders relaxed. Beginners tend to tense up the upper body around the shoulders. RELAX!

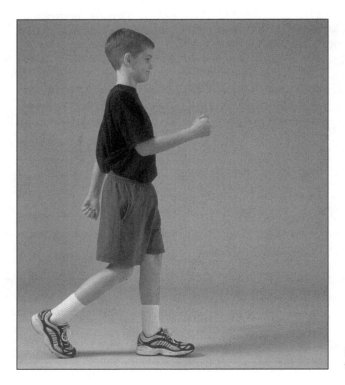

Figure 24.1 Fitness walking.

2. **Hands:** Form a loose fist. Do not clench your fist and put tension in the arm muscles.

3. **Foot placement and toe-off:** The power of the step comes from the toe-off action of the foot. With each step, land the foot on the heel, then roll forward to the toe and push off.

c. Tell the students that the above information should help them to enjoy their walking more. They should do what feels comfortable for them. DO IT RIGHT, but make it FUN!

4. The Fitness Walk

Component 1: Finding a Pulse

On the first day (or however often you would like), remind students that their pulse rate will increase when they exercise and teach them how to find their pulse.

Explain the following: During an aerobic workout, you want your heart, lungs, and blood vessels to work harder than they are used to. Your pulse can help you know what is going on inside your body. On the side of your neck just below the jaw bone is a major blood vessel bringing blood to the brain. Put your index finger and middle finger together and place them gently on that blood vessel on the side of your neck to feel the pulse. During exercise, the pulse is usually very easy to find. (To see the change in the pulse rate from the warm-up to the fitness activity to the cool-down, it would be helpful for the students to try to feel their pulse before, during, and after aerobic walking.)

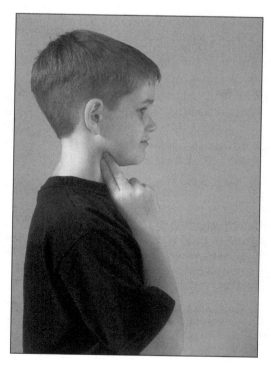

Figure 24.2 Finding your pulse.

The heart is a muscle that has a huge job to do. It must always be working, every second, minute, hour, day, week, month, and year of your lives. Once you understand that this heart muscle of yours has such a *huge* job to do, then hopefully you will want to take care of it so it can do its job.

Walking is one way to keep the heart muscle healthy. Likewise, eating right and being active are both a big part of helping the heart stay healthy. If the heart is working harder than it's used to (feel the pulse) during the fitness activity, then with time the heart will get stronger and stay healthy. The more you include exercise and eating right in your daily lives, the better the body can work and feel!

Component 2: The Safe Workout

Step 1: The warm-up. Start each fitness walk with a slow walk to get the body ready. Emphasize to students the importance of warming-up and stretching before doing any type of physical activity. During the warm-up, talk about the "adventure" for the day. Review the important facts about the warm-up. (Refer to lesson 3, "The Safe Workout: An Introduction.")

Step 2: The stretch. After the warm-up, stretch out and work on flexibility fitness. Review the importance of stretching and the key parts of safe stretching.

Step 3: Fitness activity. Introduce the fitness-walking activity you have chosen for your class, such as walking the first leg of a trip across the U.S. Have the class set a goal for that particular day. For example, the goal for the first day may be for the class to walk for five minutes without stopping. As students get used to the program, the class can set goals to walk longer and more frequently. Remember, the more days students walk, the greater the opportunity they have to learn and the more fit they will become.

Take the students on their fitness walk. During the walk, lead a discussion among students about the geographic region they are "walking through" on their program. Other topics to discuss may include nutrition and physical activity issues.

Step 4: Cool-down. After their fitness walk, have students walk more slowly to let their bodies recover.

Step 5: Cool-down stretch. After the cool-down, have students stretch out again to prevent soreness, to improve flexibility, and to decrease their chances of injury.

Step 6: The stay healthy corner. After the first walk, gather the class together and review the benefits of walking. Stress the importance of walking and the enjoyment they will gain from it. Introduce the classroom walking logs and fill them out together. Introduce and fill out together the classroom walking logs—worksheet #1, "Teacher Classroom Walking Log" and worksheet #2, "Student Classroom Walking Log."

Introduce and distribute worksheet #3, "Student Home Walking Log," to students. Review with them the four parts of the log sheet—(1) Date, (2) Time, (3) Miles, (4) Where—and how to complete it.

You and your students can decide how to use the home walking log. For example, students can keep track of their after-school walking program completely on their own, including tracking their progress on separate maps. Or students can integrate their after-school walking experience with their in-school tracking system.

However you approach it, the ultimate goal is to encourage and motivate students to exercise at home with family and/or friends.

Teacher Classroom Walking Log

Name_____ Class_____

Our fitness walk will take us across _____

_____

Table 24.1   Teacher Classroom Walking Log

Date	Time	Miles	Where

Date: Date of the fitness walk

Time: Number of minutes walked

Miles: Number of miles walked (depends on how many minutes your class decided equals one mile)

Where: Town, city, state, or country traveled through today

Student Classroom Walking Log

Name_____ Class_____

Our fitness walk will take us across _____

_____

Table 24.2   Student Classroom Walking Log

Date	Time	Miles	Where

Date: Date of the fitness walk

Time: Number of minutes walked

Miles: Number of miles walked (depends on how many minutes your class decided equals one mile)

Where: Town, city, state, or country traveled through today

Student Home Walking Log

Name _____ Class _____

My fitness walk will take me across _____

_____

Table 24.3   Student Home Walking Log

Date	Time	Miles	Where

Date: Date of the fitness walk

Time: Number of minutes walked

Miles: Number of miles walked (depends on how many minutes your class decided equals one mile)

Where: Town, city, state, or country traveled through today

Promotions for the Classroom

Part III includes four promotions that further reinforce the messages of the fourth- and fifth-grade classroom lessons and provide students an engaging opportunity to put their nutrition and physical activity knowledge into practice. *Freeze My TV* focuses on limiting television viewing. Get 3-at-School & 5-A-Day encourages students to get enough fruits and vegetables. Class-Walking Clubs offer a fun way to work regular activity into the school day, and the Pyramid Power Game reviews the messages of the Food Guide Pyramid.

As with most parts of Eat Well & *Keep Moving,* the promotions can be successfully used on their own but are most powerful when combined with the classroom lessons and other Eat Well & *Keep Moving* activities.

- *Freeze My TV* is an activity where students keep track of and try to limit the amount of television they watch for an entire week. In addition to keeping track of the time they spend watching television, students also complete graphing activities, answer questions based on their graphs, and make entries each day in the *Freeze My TV Journal.*

- Get 3-at-School & 5-A-Day allows students to put their knowledge of healthful eating into practice by trying to consume at least three servings of fruits and vegetables while at school. Each student tracks his or her at-school fruit and vegetable consumption on a large class graph. In addition to getting three servings of fruits and vegetables while at school, students are also encouraged to get a total of five servings for the entire day.

- The Class-Walking Clubs encourage classes to chart walking routes around their school and to go on walks with their teacher at least once a week. To add interest to the club, classes are encouraged to "walk" across a part of the world. Each time they walk, they can accrue a certain number of miles and mark their progress on a map.

- The Pyramid Power Game turns the messages of the Food Guide Pyramid into a fun and edifying board game. Played in groups or as an entire class, the Pyramid Power Game can serve as a daily review for the classroom and physical education lessons as well as a refresher of the Eat Well & *Keep Moving* messages throughout the school year. The game consists of a set of question cards and a Food Guide Pyramid board depicting the number of recommended servings for each food group. When students answer the nutrition-related questions on the cards correctly, they receive points that go toward filling in the recommended servings on the pyramid game board. The first student or group to fill in all the servings wins the game.

Freeze My TV

Background

Freeze My TV, an extension activity to Eat Well & *Keep Moving*'s lesson 8 and lesson 19, challenges students to keep track of and limit the amount of time they spend watching television in a designated week.

For each day of an entire seven-day week, students will log the number of hours they spend viewing television, watching videotapes, and playing video games. By keeping track of their own viewing habits, students can then see how they compare to other youth their age, as well as to the American Academy of Pediatrics' recommended goal of watching no more than two hours of television per day.

In addition to logging time spent viewing television, students will engage in other activities such as graphing, making charts, and writing in journals.

Objectives

1. To have fourth- and fifth-grade students spend a week keeping track of their time spent viewing television and to apply this information and experience to making graphs and writing in a journal.

2. To have fourth- and fifth-grade students try to limit their time spent viewing television to no more than two hours each day.

3. To have students generate alternative ways (especially physically active ways) to spend their time other than watching television. Examples are dancing, playing a game, moving around, helping with chores or doing a puzzle, reading, talking with friends, singing, writing songs or poems.

Materials

Freeze My TV packet (Television Viewing Chart; Graph-It Worksheet; Graph-It Questions; and the *Freeze My TV Journal*), Contest Participant Check List.

Procedure

1. *Freeze My TV* may be run in conjunction with the Eat Well & *Keep Moving*'s grade 4 lesson 8 and grade 5 lesson 19. This is not a necessity, however. You also may run the activity independently from the lessons, if this works better with the class schedule. Another option is to run the promotion multiple times throughout the school year to rate changes in students' TV-viewing behavior.

2. Distribute the *Freeze My TV* packet to students (provide one packet for each student) and review the materials.

3. Have students take the Television Viewing Chart home and keep track of the number of hours of television they watch each day for an entire seven-day week.

4. Tell students that their goal for the week is to limit their viewing of television to two hours or less each day, and that the class will keep a chart so that they can see how they are all doing with the goal.

5. Each day, have students report how much television they watched the day before, and record this onto a large class chart. Encourage students who watched more than two hours of television to watch less the next day.

6. After each day of trying to limit their television viewing, have students write an entry in the *Freeze My TV Journal.* Suggested topics for each day's entry appear in the journal.

7. Remind students that even if they are absent from school, they still need to keep track of their TV time and make entries in their journals.

8. At the end of the seven days, have students complete the graphing activities and questions on the Graph-It worksheets.

9. Review worksheets with students.

10. Complete the Contest Participant Check List.

Tip: One easy way for students to cut down on television time is to take the TV out of the room where they sleep (if applicable). If they don't want to physically take the TV out of the room, then they can just unplug it.

Prizes

If you have access to small giveaways, all students who complete the entire Television Viewing Chart, the Graph-It worksheets, and the *Freeze My TV Journal* can be part of a drawing to win small prizes.

Television Viewing Chart

1. Your goal for *Freeze MyTV* is to try and cut back on the amount of TV you watch for an entire week. It is best to watch no more than two hours of TV a day, and less would be even better. See how you can do compared to your classmates.

2. Have your chart with you every time you watch television (including watching TV at a friend or relative's house).

3. Each time you sit down to watch television, watch a videotape, or play a computer game that uses the television (like Nintendo), write down how much time you spent. To be sure of the time, mark down the time you started watching the television (remember to include videos and computer games) and the time you stopped.

4. At the end of each day, add up the number of hours you watched television that day. At the end of the week, add up the number of hours for the week.

5. Bring this chart with you to school each day.

EXAMPLE:

Day of the Week	Time started watching TV or playing video games	Time stopped watching TV or playing video games	Total time watched
Monday			
Morning	7:00 A.M.	8:00 A.M.	1.0 hour
Afternoon	3:00 P.M.	3:30 P.M.	0.5 hour
Evening	8:00 P.M.	9:00 P.M.	1.0 hour
		Total time for day:	2.5 hours

Teacher Example Sheet

Television Viewing Chart

Name: _____   **Date started:** _____

Day of the Week	Time started watching TV or playing video games	Time stopped watching TV or playing video games	Total time watched
_____ Morning Afternoon Evening	_____ _____ _____	_____ _____ _____	_____ _____ _____
		Total time for day:	_____
_____ Morning Afternoon Evening	_____ _____ _____	_____ _____ _____	_____ _____ _____
		Total time for day:	_____
_____ Morning Afternoon Evening	_____ _____ _____	_____ _____ _____	_____ _____ _____
		Total time for day:	_____
_____ Morning Afternoon Evening	_____ _____ _____	_____ _____ _____	_____ _____ _____
		Total time for day:	_____

Day of the Week	Time started watching TV or playing video games	Time stopped watching TV or playing video games	Total time watched
Morning Afternoon Evening			
		Total time for day:	
Morning Afternoon Evening			
		Total time for day:	
Morning Afternoon Evening			
		Total time for day:	
		Weekly total:	

Graph-It Worksheet

Name_____ Date_____

1. Using the information from the Television Viewing Chart, graph the number of hours you spent watching television each day.

2. Using the information from the Television Viewing Chart, create a graph which compares the number of hours you spent watching television each day with the daily two-hour goal during the *Freeze My TV* Week.

3. Create a graph comparing the total number of hours you spent viewing television for the entire week and the maximum number of hours per week you should watch based on the two hours per day recommendation.

4. Create a graph comparing the total number of hours you spent viewing television for the entire week and the total number of hours you spent in school for the entire week.

Worksheet 1

Graph-It Questions

1. Were you able to reach the *Freeze My TV* goal of watching less than two hours of television on any of the days? Were you able to reach the goal for the entire week? How much over or under the goal were you?

   _____

   _____

   _____

   _____

2. What activities did you do instead of watching television? Which of these activities did you enjoy most? Which were active (kept you moving around)?

   _____

   _____

   _____

   _____

3. Do you think you spent a lot of time watching TV compared to being at school? What do you think about this?

   _____

   _____

   _____

   _____

4. **Extra Credit:**

   About how much time have you spent watching TV in your lifetime? How did you figure this out? Explain your answer.

   _____

   _____

   _____

   _____

Teacher Example Sheet

Graph-It Worksheet Completed

Name_____ Date_____

1. Using the information from the Television Viewing Chart, graph the number of hours you spent watching television each day.

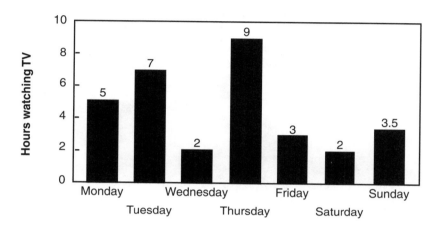

Days of the week

2. Using the information from the Television Viewing Chart, create a graph which compares the number of hours you spent watching television each day with the daily two-hour goal during the *Freeze My TV* Week.

Example #1

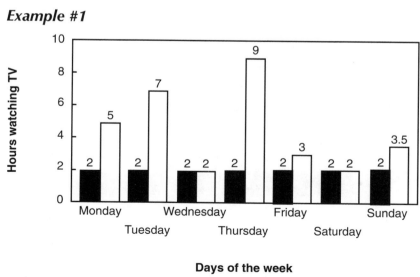

Days of the week

| ■ 2 hour per day recommendation | □ TV time |

Example #2

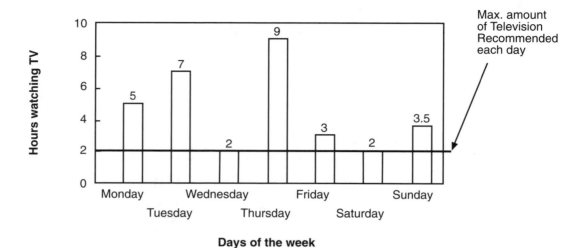

3. Create a graph comparing the total number of hours you spent viewing television for the entire week and the maximum number of hours per week you should watch based on the two hours per day recommendation.

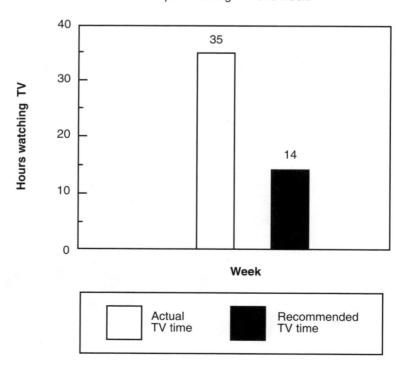

4. Create a graph comparing the total number of hours you spent viewing television for the entire week and the total number of hours you spent in school for the entire week.

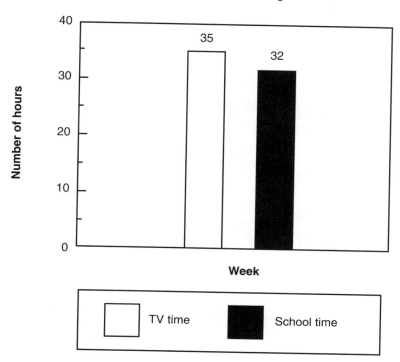

Total hours for a week spent
in school and viewing TV.

Graph-It Questions

1. Were you able to reach the *Freeze My TV* goal of watching less than two hours of television on any of the days? Were you able to reach the goal for the entire week? How much over or under the goal were you?

2. What activities did you do instead of watching television? Which of these activities did you enjoy most? Which were active (kept you moving around)?

3. Do you think you spent a lot of time watching TV compared to being at school? What do you think about this?

4. *Extra Credit:*

   About how much time have you spent watching TV in your lifetime? How did you figure this out? Explain your answer.

Teacher Example of
Contest Participant Check List

Teacher _____

School _____ Grade _____

Dates of contest: Started _____ Concluded _____

Student name	Television Tracking Chart	Graph-It Worksheet	Freeze My TV Journal
1.	Completed ❏	Completed ❏	Completed ❏
2.	Completed ❏	Completed ❏	Completed ❏
3.	Completed ❏	Completed ❏	Completed ❏
4.	Completed ❏	Completed ❏	Completed ❏
5.	Completed ❏	Completed ❏	Completed ❏
6.	Completed ❏	Completed ❏	Completed ❏
7.	Completed ❏	Completed ❏	Completed ❏
8.	Completed ❏	Completed ❏	Completed ❏
9.	Completed ❏	Completed ❏	Completed ❏
10.	Completed ❏	Completed ❏	Completed ❏
11.	Completed ❏	Completed ❏	Completed ❏
12.	Completed ❏	Completed ❏	Completed ❏
13.	Completed ❏	Completed ❏	Completed ❏
14.	Completed ❏	Completed ❏	Completed ❏
15.	Completed ❏	Completed ❏	Completed ❏
16.	Completed ❏	Completed ❏	Completed ❏
17.	Completed ❏	Completed ❏	Completed ❏
18.	Completed ❏	Completed ❏	Completed ❏
19.	Completed ❏	Completed ❏	Completed ❏
20.	Completed ❏	Completed ❏	Completed ❏

Student name	Television Tracking Chart	Graph-It Worksheet	*Freeze My TV* Journal
21.	Completed ❏	Completed ❏	Completed ❏
22.	Completed ❏	Completed ❏	Completed ❏
23.	Completed ❏	Completed ❏	Completed ❏
24.	Completed ❏	Completed ❏	Completed ❏
25.	Completed ❏	Completed ❏	Completed ❏
26.	Completed ❏	Completed ❏	Completed ❏
27.	Completed ❏	Completed ❏	Completed ❏
28.	Completed ❏	Completed ❏	Completed ❏
29.	Completed ❏	Completed ❏	Completed ❏
30.	Completed ❏	Completed ❏	Completed ❏
31.	Completed ❏	Completed ❏	Completed ❏
32.	Completed ❏	Completed ❏	Completed ❏
33.	Completed ❏	Completed ❏	Completed ❏
34.	Completed ❏	Completed ❏	Completed ❏
35.	Completed ❏	Completed ❏	Completed ❏
36.	Completed ❏	Completed ❏	Completed ❏
37.	Completed ❏	Completed ❏	Completed ❏
38.	Completed ❏	Completed ❏	Completed ❏

Please complete and return to Teacher by _____

Instructions for Assembling the Freeze My TV Journal

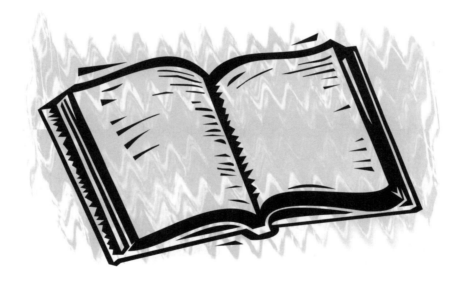

When completed, the *Freeze My TV Journal* will look like a booklet.
To do this:

1. Line up the dots that appear in the corner of every sheet so that they are all in the same corner. Some sheets will be inverted.
2. Place this packet into the photocopier and make double-sided copies of the packet.
3. Fold the packet on the dotted line.

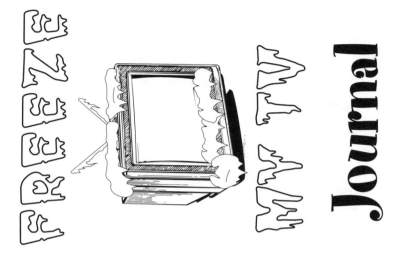

FREEZE MY TV

Journal

Fold here to make booklet.

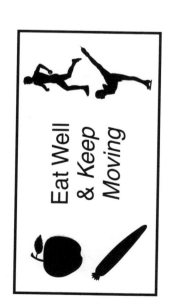

Eat Well & Keep Moving

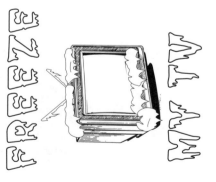

FREEZE MY TV

Name _____

Instructions

For each day of *Freeze My TV*, write a paragraph in the journal. Be sure to read the instructions for each day before you start writing.

TV Alternatives

Acting
Baby-sitting
Baseball
Basketball
Bike riding
Board games
Bowling
Camping
Capture the flag
Checkers
Chess
Cleaning the house
Computer work
Cooking
Dancing
Doing each other's hair
Drawing
Fishing
Four-square
Frisbee
Grocery shopping
Gym
Gymnastics
Hackey sack
Hide and go seek

Hiking
Hockey
Hopscotch
Invite friends over
Jogging
Jump rope
Kickball
Lacrosse
Laundry
Legos
Listening to music
Museum
Painting
Planting flowers
Playing an instrument
Pull-ups
Reading
Roller skating
Singing
Sit-ups
Skipping
Stretching
Tag
Swimming
Studying

Day 1

Date _____

Write a paragraph describing how you feel about trying to decrease the amount of television you watch for an entire week.

_____

_____

_____

_____

_____

_____

_____

_____

Day 7

Date _____

A friend of yours wants to try to watch less television. Write a paragraph to him/her with some tips that helped you cut back on watching TV.

_____
_____
_____
_____
_____
_____
_____
_____
_____

Day 2

Date _____

Write a paragraph describing what day 1 of *Freeze My TV* week was like. Did you like watching less television? Did you not like watching less television?

_____
_____
_____
_____
_____
_____
_____
_____
_____

Day 3

Date _____

Write a paragraph about what you did during day 1 and day 2 when you weren't watching television. How do you think you will spend this time for the rest of the week?

_____

_____

_____

_____

_____

_____

_____

_____

_____

Day 6

Date _____

Have you missed watching all the television you usually watch? Why or why not?

_____

_____

_____

_____

_____

_____

_____

_____

_____

Day 4
Date
_____

Do you like to eat food while you watch television? If yes, what kind of food do you like to eat? Name some healthy snacks you could eat (or already eat) while watching television?

_____
_____
_____
_____
_____
_____
_____
_____

Day 5
Date
_____

Write a paragraph describing what you think people did for entertainment before television was invented? How do you think they spent their time without television?

_____
_____
_____
_____
_____
_____
_____
_____

Get 3-at-School & 5-A-Day

Background

Get 3-at-School & 5-A-Day is an activity for students that encourages them to eat at least five servings of fruits and vegetables each day—with a particular focus on getting three servings of fruits and vegetables during school breakfast and lunch. The activity reinforces, in an educational and engaging manner, many of the nutrition messages students have been exposed to as part of Eat Well & *Keep Moving* throughout the year.

Length of Activity

The activity runs for an entire school week, beginning on a Monday and ending on a Friday.

Goal

To help students think about and put into practice the 5-A-Day fruit and vegetable recommendation they have been exposed to in the classroom and cafeteria.

Materials

- Large Class Tracking Graph (example provided)
- Dole Foods "How'd You Do Your 5 Today?" chart for each student (available free from Dole Foods—see order form on p. 305)
- Dole Foods "Fun With Fruits and Vegetables Kids Cookbook" for each student (available from Dole Foods) or other cookbooks from the Produce for Better Health Foundation (**www.5aday.com**)
- Group Tracking Chart
- Eat Well cards (black and white copies are included in the appendix, pp. 460-477)
- Optional: Dole Foods "Jammin' 5-A-Day Songs" (single copies available for free to elementary school educators from the Produce for Better Health Foundation; **www.5aday.com**)

Procedure

Preparation Day

1. On Monday, announce to students that they will be taking part in a fruits and vegetables activity over the next four days (Tuesday-Friday). Provide students with an overview of the activity. Their goal is to eat three servings of fruits and vegetables every day at school (including school lunch and breakfast). They will keep track of the servings they eat on a class chart; and they will try to get at least two additional servings of fruits and vegetables outside of school so that they get a total of five for the entire day.

2. Review with students the "5-A-Day" Eat Well card (p. 462). Remind students of the benefits of eating fruits and vegetables. Highlight that fruit provides energy for playing and growing and can help their bodies heal cuts and bruises. Likewise, let them know that vegetables can help them fight infections and see better at night.

3. Create a Large Class Tracking Graph (see example on page 306).

Day 1

1. Before lunch, divide students into small groups and distribute the Group Tracking Charts (page 307). Explain that the students in each group will help each other keep track of the fruits and vegetables they eat at lunch. (Activity may also be done individually.)

2. Also before lunch, discuss with students the "What a Treat to Eat a Sweet Peach" Eat Well card.

   Note: The Eat Well cards listed for each day are only recommendations. There may be more appropriate Eat Well cards for your Get 3-at-School & 5-A-Day week—such as those that correspond to the lunch menu. You can get a copy of the menu from the cafeteria manager and determine which of the Eat Well cards (in the appendix) would work well with the lunch for each day.

3. After lunch, have the groups write down on the Group Tracking Chart the number of servings of fruits and vegetables each individual in the group ate. Remind students that they may also count any fruits or vegetables they ate for breakfast (at school or home). Remind students that fried potatoes (such as French fries and potato chips) do not count toward the 3-at-School goal, but 100% juice does (see related Eat Well card).

   Note: One "serving" can be defined as any time a student consumes the entire amount of a fruit or vegetable served to him or her in the cafeteria. If a student consumes only part of the fruit or vegetable served, it can count as a half serving. If a student just tastes a fruit or vegetable, it can count as a quarter serving. A glass of 100% juice counts as a serving.

4. Mark the students' progress on the Large Class Tracking Graph (see example). You are encouraged to track your consumption along with that of your students.

5. Explain to students that they should not stop eating fruits and vegetables once they reach the 3-at-School goal. It is important that they strive to get a total of at least five servings of fruits and vegetables each day.

6. Distribute a Dole Foods "How'd You Do Your 5 Today?" chart to each student and tell students that this chart can help them make sure they get a total of five servings for each day. Explain to students how to use the Dole tracking chart and encourage them to use the charts at home.

Day 2

1. Before lunch, discuss with students the "Potatoes" Eat Well card.

2. After lunch, have the groups write down on the Group Tracking Chart the number of servings of fruits and vegetables each individual in the group ate. Remind students that they may also count any fruits or vegetables they ate for breakfast (at school or home).

3. Mark the students' progress on the Large Class Tracking Graph.

4. Remind students that they should not stop eating fruits and vegetables once they reach the 3-at-School goal. It is important that they strive to get a total of at least five servings of fruits and vegetables each day.

Day 3

1. Before lunch, discuss with students the "A Juicy Quiz" Eat Well card. This card may be introduced by asking students who had 100% orange juice for breakfast today.

2. After lunch, have the groups write down on the Group Tracking Chart the number of servings of fruits and vegetables each individual in the group ate. Remind students that they may also count any fruits or vegetables they ate for breakfast (at school or home).

3. Mark the students' progress on the Large Class Tracking Graph.

4. Remind students that they should not stop eating fruits and vegetables once they reach the 3-at-School goal. It is important that they strive to get a total of at least five servings of fruits and vegetables each day.

The Final Day—Day 4

1. Discuss with students before lunch the "A Message from Bobby Broccoli" Eat Well card.

2. After lunch, have the groups write down on the Group Tracking Chart the number of servings of fruits and vegetables each individual in the group ate. Remind students that they may also count any fruits or vegetables they ate for breakfast (at school or home).

3. After lunch, complete the Large Class Tracking Graph and review the final results with students.

4. Remind students that eating their fruits and vegetables at lunch and getting at least five servings each day is very important for their health and will give them the energy they need to think, run, and play.

As a prize for participation, distribute to each student a Dole Foods "Fun with Fruits and Vegetables Kids Cookbook." Explain that they may want to try these recipes at home with the help of their parents or other family members.

Eat Well Cards

To complement the fruits and vegetables activity, these Eat Well cards may be discussed with students right before they go off to lunch on each day of the activity. A black and white copy of each is provided in the appendix.

Eat Well Cards Schedule

Review with students just prior to lunch.

- **Monday:** Preparation Day, 5-A-Day Should Be Your Goal
- **Tuesday:** Day 1, What a Treat to Eat a Sweet Peach
- **Wednesday:** Day 2, Potatoes
- **Thursday:** Day 3, A Juicy Quiz
- **Friday:** Day 4, A Message from Bobby Broccoli

"Jammin' 5-A-Day Songs" Audio Cassette

Dole Foods's "Jammin' 5-A-Day Songs" contains catchy songs about fruits and vegetables. The cassette is available free to elementary school educators from Dole Foods and could be played in the classroom and cafeteria during the Get 3-at-School & 5-A-Day activity.

On school letterhead, fax a request for a single copy of the cassette to Dole Foods (415-570-5250). Include teacher name, school address, and phone number. Visit **www.dole5aday.com** for more information.

Free 5-A-Day Materials from Dole Foods

The "Fun With Fruits and Vegetables Kids Cookbook" and 5-A-Day Tracking Chart are available free to schools.

On school letterhead, teachers should fax their name, school name and address, phone number, class size, and number of cookbooks and charts they need to 415-570-5250. Ordering information is also available at the Dole Foods 5-A-Day Web site (**http://www.dole5aday.com**). Allow at least 4 weeks for delivery.

Dole Fun With Fruits and Vegetables Kids Cookbook and How'd You Do Your 5 Today Chart Order Form

Fax form on school letterhead to: 415-570-5250

Name _____

School _____

Address _____

_____

_____

Telephone number _____

Grade Level: _____   Class Size: _____

Cookbooks: _____   # Charts: _____

More information at the Dole Web site: **www.dole5aday.com**

Large Class Tracking Graph

Example

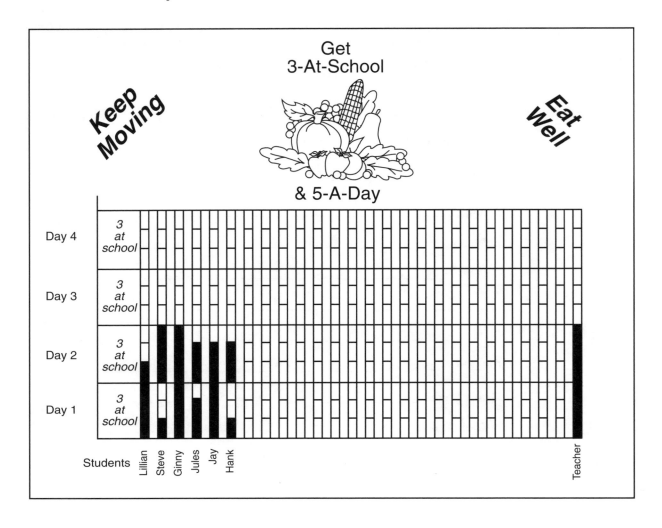

Table 26.1 Group Tracking Chart

School _____ Grade _____

Teacher _____

Group Name _____

Group Members	Servings Day 1	Servings Day 2	Servings Day 3	Servings Day 4	Total Servings

Class-Walking Clubs

Background

This document describes how you can begin an ongoing walking club with your students. Not only will such a walking club be fun and healthful for your students it will also be educational.

Note: This description also appears as part of the Fitness Walking lessons (lesson 12 in grade 4 and lesson 24 in grade 5) in the Eat Well & *Keep Moving* grade 4 and grade 5 lesson-set.

Objectives

1. For students to participate regularly in a walking activity and to establish an ongoing class walking club
2. For students to learn about the benefits of walking with family, friends, and classmates
3. For students to learn walking techniques and the health benefits of raising one's heart rate through regular aerobic activity
4. For students to learn about a particular geographic region of the world

Materials

1. Comfortable shoes (students and teacher)
2. Worksheet #1, "Teacher Classroom Walking Log"
3. Worksheet #2, "Student Classroom Walking Log" (duplicate for students)
4. Worksheet #3, "Student Home Walking Log" (duplicate for students)
5. Map(s)
6. Map pins/thumb tacks

Why Walking?

Walking is one of the healthiest, safest, and easiest ways to begin a fitness program and can be a big step toward improving your health. Fitness or aerobic walking uses all of the major muscle groups in the upper and lower body in a nonimpacting, dynamic, rhythmic action, which is what an ideal exercise should do.

Walking is also free! There are no machines or membership fees, no fancy packaging or expensive clothes. Walking requires only that you "race" yourself and do your "personal best." What's important is feeling good about yourself and setting your own standards and goals.

Walking can be done with friends or family. It can also be done as an adventure with a school class. An active lifestyle can make you feel better, give you more energy, and enhance your health. We want you and your class to get hooked on walking. It's fun, and it's good for you!

Planning a Walking Club

When planning a walking club, first consider where and when your students can walk. The walks can take place before, during, or after school, and can be done in the hallways, gym, playgrounds, or around the neighborhood—whenever and wherever such a program works best for your school.

An effective way to introduce a walking club into your school would be to integrate it with your curriculum. One option is to integrate the club with your social studies curriculum, for example, with lessons on the state in which you live, the entire United States, or other countries around the world. If there is an area of the world your students would like to learn about, use the walking club to help you accomplish this. As a class or individually, design the itinerary of a fitness walk across the region you have chosen to cover. Students could walk across America together, walk across a region of the U.S., or walk around the world. The design is completely open.

Give your program a name, such as "Walk Across America" or "Walk Across the World," or let the students choose a name.

Using maps of the area(s) you choose, tie in the students' walking progress with movement on the map. Each time the class walks a certain period of time, equate that with a particular distance on the map (for example, five minutes walked could equal 50 miles). Each student can have a map, or all of the students can plot their travels on one map. The amount of time the class walks and the distance traveled will depend on the part of the world or country on which you chose to focus. For example, if you decide on a large area of the world, such as Africa, then five minutes might equal 200 miles traveled. If you chose the state of Maryland, five minutes might equal 50 miles.

Keep track of your class walks on the logs provided. There is a log for each class, as well as for each student. The class log can be made larger and displayed in the classroom for all to see. A map of the area/region/country that they will be traveling across should be displayed along with the log. Displaying the map and log will motivate the class and keep everyone more involved.

Extension Ideas

As an extension of the class walking club, encourage students to take the walking club idea home, as an after-school family-or-friend adventure. Have the students keep a log of their dates and times for after-school walks (see "Student Home Walking Log" on page 317). They can plot their travels on the maps with pins or thumb tacks.

Get the whole school involved in walking—principals, office staff, custodians, and other teachers and students can become involved. The more the students see others participating, the more they will want to become involved.

Day 1

1. What Is Fitness Walking?

Explain to students that "fitness walking" is walking at a pace (speed) that makes the heart, lungs, and blood vessels work harder than usual. This type of aerobic workout makes the heart muscle pump harder because the body's other muscles—leg and arm muscles—are working harder and need more blood to keep them going.

Blood gives muscles energy to work. When muscles work hard, such as when you're doing fitness walking, they need more energy. During exercise, the heart works harder to pump blood to these muscles. When the heart works hard, it gets stronger.

Explain to students that they can check their pulse rate before they begin exercising and again during their fitness workout in order to see firsthand how the heart muscle works harder. (See details on how to do this in the section "Finding a Pulse".)

2. Benefits of Fitness Walking

Ask students to list the benefits of fitness walking. These can include the following:

a. Walking is an excellent and safe way to achieve aerobic conditioning. Aerobic conditioning means taking care of the heart, lungs, and blood vessels. Walking lets you do this with less wear and tear on the body compared to many other types of conditioning.

b. Walking and other aerobic exercises can give you more energy and reduce fatigue.

c. Walking can help relieve stress.

d. Walking can improve mood and mental function.

e. Walking can help in weight control.

f. Walking can help slow down the progression of osteoporosis (bone loss), which can occur when one ages.

g. Walking can be performed with friends and family.

3. How to Fitness Walk

a. Make sure students wear sneakers or comfortable shoes.

b. Review with students the following:

1. **Arm swing:** Try to keep the arms swinging at a pace faster than they swing when walking normally. The faster the arms swing, the faster the legs will move. Bend the arms 90 degrees at the elbow. Concentrate on moving the arms faster and swinging them from the shoulder. Remember, when you shorten your arms (bending them at the elbow 90 degrees), you can swing them faster and your legs will move faster. Keep your shoulders relaxed. Beginners tend to tense up the upper body around the shoulders. RELAX!

2. **Hands:** Form a loose fist. Do not clench your fist and put tension in the arm muscles.

3. **Foot placement and toe-off:** The power of the step comes from the toe-off action of the foot. With each step, land the foot on the heel, then roll forward to the toe and push off.

c. Tell the students the above information should help them to enjoy their walking more. They should do what feels comfortable for them. DO IT RIGHT, but make it FUN!

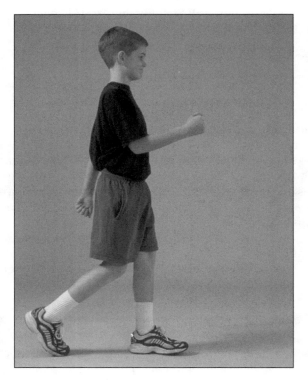

Figure 27.1 Fitness walking.

4. The Fitness Walk

Step 1: Finding a Pulse

On the first day (or however often you would like), remind students that their pulse rate will increase when they exercise and teach the students how to find their pulse.

Explain the following: During an aerobic workout, you want your heart, lungs, and blood vessels to work harder than they are used to. Your pulse can help you know what is going on inside your body. On the side of your neck just below the jaw bone is a major blood vessel bringing blood to the brain. Put your index finger and middle finger together and place them gently on that blood vessel on the side of your neck to feel the pulse. During exercise, the pulse is usually very easy to find. (To see the change in the pulse rate from the warm-up to the fitness activity to the cool-down, it would be helpful for the students to try to feel their pulse before, during, and after aerobic walking.)

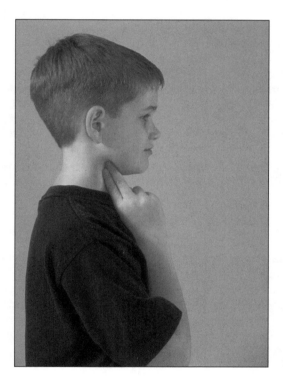

Figure 27.2   Finding your pulse.

The heart is a muscle that has a huge job to do. It must always be working, every second, minute, hour, day, week, month, and year of your lives. Once you understand that this heart muscle of yours has such a *huge* job to do, then hopefully you will want to take care of it so it can do its job.

Walking is one way to keep the heart muscle healthy. Likewise, eating right and being active are both a big part of helping the heart stay healthy. If the heart is working harder than it's used to (feel the pulse) during the fitness activity, then with time the heart will get stronger and stay healthy. The more you include exercise and eating right in your daily lives, the better the body can work and feel!

Step 2: The Walk

Introduce the fitness-walking activity you have chosen for your class, such as walking the first leg of a trip across the U.S. Have the class set a goal for that particular day. For example, the goal for the first day may be for the class to walk for five minutes without stopping. As students get used to the program, the class can set goals to walk longer and more frequently. Remember, the more days students walk, the greater the opportunity they have to learn and the more fit they will become.

Start each walking session with a few minutes of slow walking to get the body warmed up. After this, the walking can get a bit faster. During the walk, lead discussion among students about the geographic region they are "walking through" on their program. Other topics may include nutrition and physical activity issues.

After their main walk, have students walk more slowly to let their bodies cool down.

If time allows, the class can also stretch after the warm-up and cool-down. Follow stretching examples in lesson 3 of the Eat Well & *Keep Moving* grade 4 lesson-set.

Step 3: The Stay Healthy Corner

After the first walk, gather the class together and review the benefits of walking. Stress the importance of walking and the enjoyment they will get from it. Introduce and fill out together the classroom walking logs—worksheet #1, "Teacher Classroom Walking Log" and worksheet #2, "Student Classroom Walking Log."

Introduce and distribute worksheet #3, "Student Home Walking Log," to students. Review with them the four parts of the log sheet—(1) Date, (2) Time, (3) Miles, (4) Where—and how to complete it.

You and your students can decide how to use worksheet #3, "Student Home Walking Log." For example, students can keep track of their after-school walking program completely on their own, including tracking their progress on separate maps. Or students can integrate their after-school walking experience with their in-school tracking system.

However you approach it, the ultimate goal is to encourage and motivate students to exercise at home with family and/or friends.

Day 2 and Beyond

The walking clubs are intended to continue throughout the school year and, whenever possible, should be done at least two to three times a week.

When the class has completed "walking" across one region, they can vote for the next region they would like to walk across. To make the activity even more interesting, the class can also "climb" a mountain—such as Mt. McKinley (Denali) or Mt. Everest—or they can "walk" between the planets in the solar system, through the center of the earth, or along the circulatory system of the body.

Teacher Classroom Walking Log

Name _____ Class _____

Our fitness walk will take us across _____
_____

Table 27.1   **Teacher Classroom Walking Log**

Date	Time	Miles	Where

Date: Date of the fitness walk

Time: Number of minutes walked

Miles: Number of miles walked (depends on how many minutes your class decided equals one mile)

Where: Town, city, state, or country traveled through today

Student Classroom Walking Log

Name_____ Class_____

Our fitness walk will take us across _____

_____

Table 27.2   Student Classroom Walking Log

Date	Time	Miles	Where

Date: Date of the fitness walk

Time: Number of minutes walked

Miles: Number of miles walked (depends on how many minutes your class decided equals one mile)

Where: Town, city, state, or country traveled through today

Student Home Walking Log

Name _____ Class _____

My fitness walk will take me across _____

_____

Table 27.3   Student Home Walking Log

Date	Time	Miles	Where

Date: Date of the fitness walk

Time: Number of minutes walked

Miles: Number of miles walked (depends on how many minutes your class decided equals one mile)

Where: Town, city, state, or country traveled through today

Pyramid Power Game

Background

The Food Guide Pyramid promotes moderation, variety, and balance in the diet and helps individuals choose what and how much to eat from each food group so they get the nutrients they need for lifelong health.

There are six categories in the pyramid, and the size of each category corresponds to the amount of food from that group that you need to eat each day. The groups toward the bottom of the pyramid take up more space, which means that you need more of these foods and less of the foods closer to the top. The food group at the tip of the pyramid contains foods high in fat and/or sugar. It is healthy to eat these only in small amounts. For instance, a diet low in saturated and *trans* fats may help reduce your risk of heart disease.

This activity may be used as an assessment for the preceding nutrition lessons.

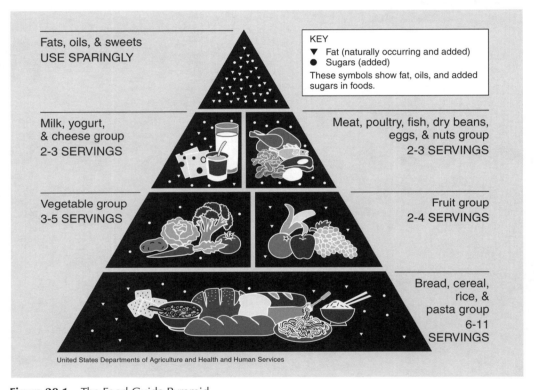

Figure 28.1 The Food Guide Pyramid.

Estimated Teaching Time and Related Subject Area

Estimated teaching time: 1 hour

Related subject area: math

Objectives

1. Students will review general knowledge of the Food Guide Pyramid.
2. Students will reinforce their factual knowledge about the Food Guide Pyramid and appropriate food choices.

Materials

1. Handout/transparency #1, "Food Guide Pyramid"
2. Game sheet #1, "Pyramid Power Game Instructions"
3. Game sheet #2, "Pyramid Power Game Board" (Size: 8 1/2" by 11") for each person in each group (excluding question reader) or one for each group, depending on method of play
4. Game sheet #3, "Game Disks/Markers" (may be cut from sheets provided)
5. Game sheet #4, "Game Cards" (to be photocopied)

Procedure

Part I

1. Display blank outline of Food Guide Pyramid. Have students recall the names of the food groups and the number of servings recommended each day. Have students record these on the pyramid outline.
2. Ask some of the students to name a food they ate yesterday. Ask the class to tell you into which food group each of the named foods goes.
3. Tell students that this information will assist them in playing the "Pyramid Power Game."

Part II

1. Explain "Pyramid Power Game" rules.
2. Show students one of the game cards and read the question.

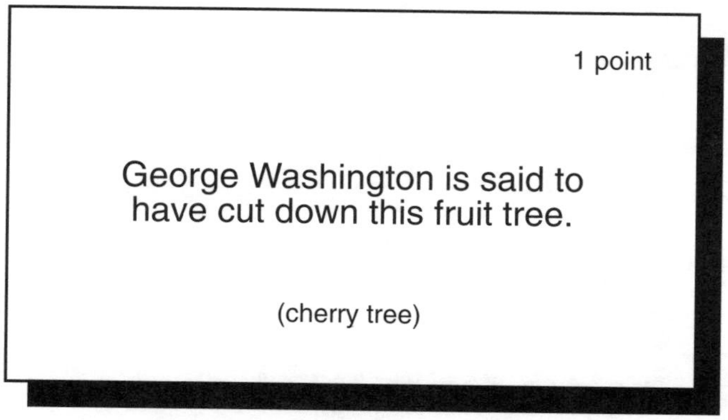

Figure 28.2 Pyramid Power Game card.

3. Have a student answer, then explain to the class what happens when a correct answer is given. (See "Pyramid Power Game Instructions.")

Part III

1. Distribute game boards, markers, and questions to each group leader.

2. Review the game rules and provide an opportunity for students to ask questions, then begin the game.

3. At the end of 15-20 minutes, if a winner is not declared, the teacher may end the game by announcing, "Last two questions coming up!" (the group with the most "servings" is the winner).

4. Review the correct answers to missed game card questions with students.

The Food Guide Pyramid

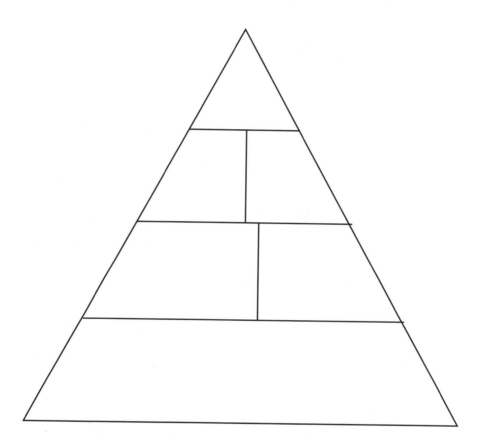

Pyramid Power Game Instructions

Purpose of the Game

In this game, students respond to questions relating to the six sections of the Food Guide Pyramid. New questions may be added by the teacher as new concepts are introduced. The game may also serve as a means of reinforcing previously taught information.

Materials

1. Game card questions for each group (to be photocopied from cards provided)
2. Game board (8 1/2" by 11") for each person in group (excluding question reader) or one for each group, depending on method of play
3. Game disks/markers (to be cut from sheet provided)

Setting Up the Game

The game questions are coded "1 point," "2 points," or "3 points" (see following pages). The teacher will need to photocopy the cards and cut them up for each group. There will be approximately 60 questions in a deck. Shuffle the deck and place face down on the top of a desk or table.

Playing the Game

Here are two ways to play the game:

Option One: Divide the class into groups of four, five, or six. Assign one person in each group to be the "question reader" and distributor of disks for the group. In this case, the members of each group compete against one another. There will be one winner from each group.

Option Two: Divide the class into groups of four, five, or six. Read the questions to the class and the members of each group work cooperatively to come up with an answer. In this case, the groups compete against each other.

The leader draws one card at a time, in order from the top, and reads the question to the group/s. Players take turns responding to questions. If the student answers correctly he/she receives one, two, or three disks, depending on the value of the question. This disk is placed on the game board in a space marked "serving," indicating one serving.

A player must accumulate enough disks (markers) to cover the minimum number of servings for each food group, beginning with the grain section. For example, six servings are represented in the grain section on the board; therefore six markers are needed to cover all grain servings before moving to the next level (fruits and vegetables).

To speed up the game, four cards marked BONUS have been added to the deck. When one of these cards is drawn, a player receives four additional bonus markers if he/she answers the question on the card correctly.

How to Win

The first player (or group) to cover all the serving spaces on the board wins the game.

Note: While the game cards include many answers to the open-ended questions, they may not include all possible answers. If students have a question about a possibly correct answer that is not included on a card, they should be encouraged to share it with you.

Pyramid Power Game Board

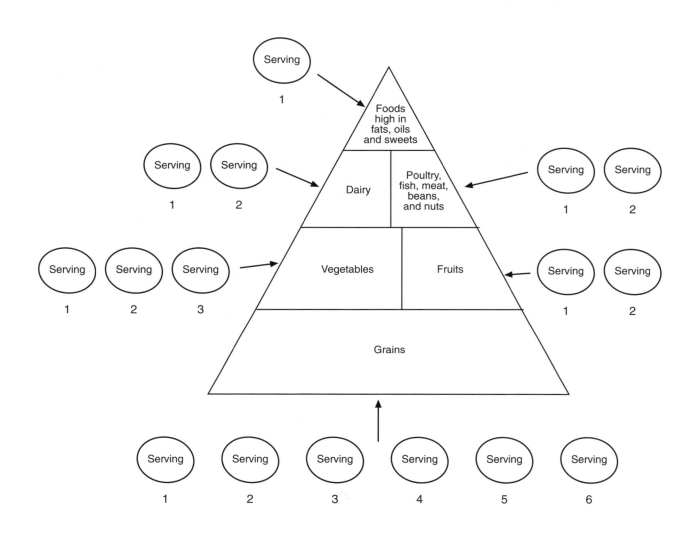

Pyramid Power
Game Disks (copy and cut out)

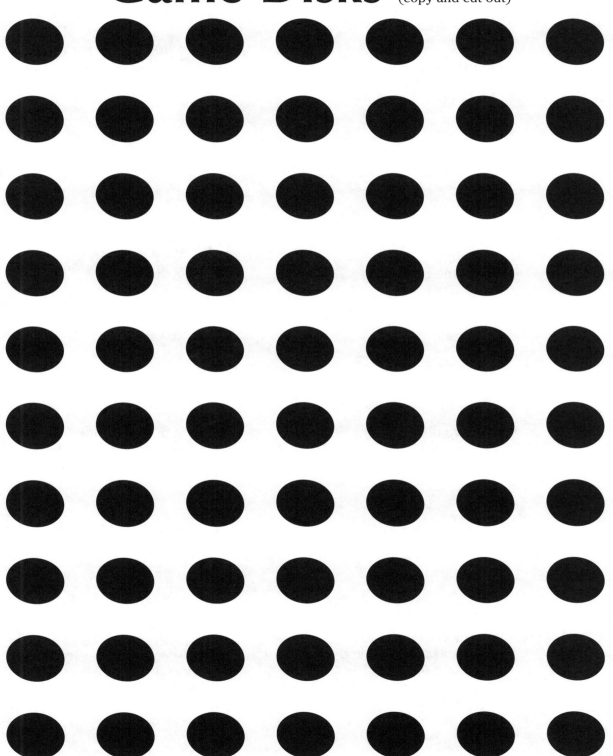

Pyramid Power Game Cards (copy and cut out)

---

1 point

Name the vegetable that Peter Rabbit got from Mr. McGregor's garden.

(cabbage)

---

1 point

Where does ice cream fit in the Food Guide Pyramid?

(the top/tip)

---

1 point

Bread comes in many different forms — name two.

(rolls, loaf, stick, pita, tortilla)

• •BONUS• •
4 points

Where does yogurt fit in the Food Guide Pyramid?

(the dairy group)

---

1 point

Name two edible nuts.

(peanut, cashew, hazelnut, Brazil, almond, macadamia)

---

1 point

Where do french fries fit in the Food Guide Pyramid?

(the top/tip)

---

1 point

Name a grain or grain food that you would probably find in a Mexican restaurant.

(corn, rice, tortilla)

---

1 point

What name is given to a person who sits and watches television for long periods of time?
Hint: based on a vegetable

(couch potato)

---

1 point

Complete the name of this famous combo:

"Red beans and _____."

(rice)

---

1 point

You should be sure to eat at least _____ servings of fruit each day.

(2)

---

1 point

Where would you find Cheerios in the Food Guide Pyramid?

(grain group)

---

1 point

How many servings of vegetables should you be sure to have each day?

(3 servings)

---

1 point

Name a doll that is named after a green vegetable.

(Cabbage Patch)

---

1 point

How many servings of bread, cereal, rice, and pasta, should you be sure to have each day?

(6 servings)

• •Bonus• •
4 points

Where would cornflakes be found in the Food Guide Pyramid?

(grain group)

---

1 point

Name three kinds of fruit you might find in a fruit cocktail.

(cherry, pear, pineaple, peach)

Gamesheet 4

---

1 point

Complete the name of
this edible flower:

_____lion

(dandelion)

---

1 point

Name a vegetable that
grows a head.

(cabbage, lettuce, cauliflower, broccoli,
brussels sprouts)

••BONUS••
4 points

Name a food that is a
good source of iron.

(spinach, meat, liver, broccoli)

---

2 points

Which food has the most iron —
liver, green beans, or corn?

(liver)

---

1 point

Name something you would
not put on popcorn if you
wanted a fat-free snack.

(butter, margarine, cheese, oil)

••BONUS••
4 points

Name a nutrient found
in orange juice.

(vitamin C, carbohydrates)

---

2 points

Name three berries with
compound names.

(strawberry, blueberry, blackberry)

---

2 points

Name two leafy,
green vegetables.

(kale, spinach, collard greens,
romaine lettuce)

---

1 point

Jack traded his cow for
what type of seeds?

(beans)

1 point

How many servings of low-fat
milk, yogurt, and cheese should
you be sure to have each day?

(2 servings)

1 point

Name an edible seed.

(sunflower, pumpkin, poppy, sesame)

1 point

Name a large, orange fruit
that is popular during
an October celebration.

(pumpkin)

1 point

Name two fruits that
grow in bunches.

(bananas, grapes)

1 point

What equals a serving of bread—
1/2 slice, 1 slice, or 2 slices?

(1 slice)

1 point

Name a fruit that
looks like a small
orange.

(tangerine, tangelo, clementine,
kumquat, persimmon)

1 point

What equals a serving
of cooked vegetables —
1/2 cup, 1 cup, or 2 cups?

(1/2 cup)

1 point

Name a fuzzy fruit.

(kiwi, peach)

---

1 point

Of the following, what best describes a healthy diet?

1. *Eating no fat at all*
2. *Eating lots of sweets*
3. *Eating a lot of different foods from all the food groups*

(#3)

---

1 point

Name a vegetable that grows as a stalk.

(rhubarb, celery)

---

1 point

What is the minumum number of servings of fruits and vegetables you should eat every day —
3, 5, or 7 servings?

(5 servings)

---

1 point

Cinderella's magic coach was made of what kind of fruit?

(pumpkin)

---

1 point

Which would be a healther food choice —
cheddar cheese or low-fat cheese

(low-fat cheese)

---

1 point

Name a large fruit with dark and light green skin and a red center with seeds.

(watermelon)

---

1 point

Which would be a healthier food choice —
bologna or turkey?

(turkey)

1 point

Name two ways
to serve carrots.

(raw or cooked)

---

1 point

Which would be a
healthier food choice —

french fries or a plain baked potato?

(plain baked potato)

---

2 points

Name a yellow vegetable
that has a "q" in its name.

(squash)

---

1 point

Which would be a
healthier snack choice —

Doritos or low-salt pretzels?

(low-salt pretzels)

---

1 point

George Washington is said
to have cut down
this fruit tree.

(cherry tree)

---

1 point

Which would be a
healthier food choice —

ice cream or low-fat frozen yogurt?

(low-fat frozen yogurt)

---

1 point

How many teaspoons of fat
are there in a McDonald's
quarter pounder with cheese —

0, 3, or 7 teaspoons?

(7 teaspoons)

---

1 point

Which would be a
healthier food choice —

baked chicken or fried chicken?

(baked chicken)

1 point

Name a food that may be
labelled "seafood."

(fish, crab, lobster, clams, shrimp,
oysters, mussels, abalone)

---

1 point

Which would be a
healthier food choice —
*pepperoni pizza or
mushroom pizza?*

(mushroom pizza)

---

1 point

Name a food that is
a type of poultry.

(chicken, turkey, duck, Cornish hen)

---

1 point

Which would be a
healthier food choice —
a donut or cereal?

(cereal)

---

2 points

Name a nut from which
a common cooking food
is extracted.

(peanut)

---

2 points

Which is better for
your health —
olive oil or lard?

(olive oil)

---

1 point

Name a food, found in the
grain group, that is served
with tomato sauce.

(pasta, rice)

---

2 points

Name one vegetable that
you would expect to find
in succotash.

(corn, lima beans)

2 points

Name the major
vitamin that you get
from citrus fruits.

(vitamin C)

---

1 point

Where would you find cake/pie
in the Food Guide Pyramid?

(the tip/top)

---

2 points

A plantain is sometimes
confused with a _____.

(banana)

---

1 point

Name a grain food that
is a part of lasagna.

(noodles, pasta)

---

2 points

What is the main
difference between a
fruit and a vegetable?

(fruits must have internal seeds)

---

2 points

Complete the name of this
popular breakfast food:

cream of _____.

(wheat)

---

1 point

How much (in terms of weight)
of a watermelon really
is water —

25%, 50%, or 90%?

(90%)

---

1 point

Which types of lettuce
are more nutritious —

light green or dark green?

(dark green)

Gamesheet

4

••BONUS••
4 points

What disease did many early explorers get from not getting enough vitamin C?

1. scurvy
2. mad cow disease
3. chicken pox

(scurvy)

---

2 points

True or false — frozen fruits and vegetables are not as good for you as fresh vegetables

(false)

---

2 points

Which of the following may happen if you don't eat enough vitamin C

1. you won't be able to find your dog
2. you'll have trouble seeing at night
3. you will get a stuffy nose

(#2)

---

2 points

True or false — A dog's body can make vitamin C but a person's body cannot.

(true)

---

1 point

Kale, collard greens, and turnip greens have a lot of:

1. fat
2. salt
3. vitamins and minerals

(#3, vitamins and minerals)

---

2 points

Name a dairy product that may be eaten with spaghetti?

(low-fat cheese, low-fat yogurt)

---

1 point

Which tends to have more nutrients —
raw vegetables or cooked vegetables

(raw vegetables)

---

1 point

How many pounds of pasta (like spaghetti and macaroni) does the average American eat each year?

1. 1 pound
2. 7 pounds
3. 20 pounds

(#3, 20 pounds)

---

2 points

Which grain is consumed the most in the United States?

1. Rice
2. Corn
3. Wheat
4. Barley

(wheat)

2 points

What do jelly, jam, and syrup have in common?

(They are found at the tip/top of the pyramid; they contain sugar; they are made from plant products)

1 point

In which group in the Food Guide Pyramid does pasta belong?

1. fruit
2. grain
3. beans, meat, and nuts
4. vegetable
5. dairy
6. fats, oils, and sweets

(grain)

1 point

Most of the food we eat should come from which Food Guide Pyramind group?

(grain group)

2 points

True or false —
a serving of 100% fruit juice counts toward your 5-a-day.

(true)

2 points

True or false —
fiber is important for good health.

(true)

2 points

True or false —
drinking enough water is very important for good health.

(true)

2 points

True or false —
one baked potato with the skin has more vitamin C than one tomato.

(true)

Gamesheet 4

---

1 point

Complete the name of
this vegetable:

Sweet _____

(potato, corn, basil, peas)

---

3 points

What does the phrase "empty
calories" mean?

1. *a food has no calories*
2. *a food provides only calories*
and little or no vitamins or minerals

(#2, it means that a food provides no
vitamins and minerals, only calories)

---

2 points

True or false —
food gives us the calories
we need to live, study,
work, and play.

(true)

---

3 points

How many calories does
1 gram of fat provide?

(9 calories per gram)

---

3 points

How many calories does
1 gram of protein provide?

(4 calories per gram)

---

3 points

How many
calories does 1 gram of
carbohydrates provide?

(4 calories per gram)

---

1 point

Name a fruit that contains
a lot of vitamin C.

(orange, grapefruit, lemon,
strawberry, tangerine)

---

2 points

True or false —
Fats that are liquid at room
temperature (such as canola oil)
are better for your health than
fats that are solid at room
temperature (such as butter).

(true)

---

2 points

Name a long, orange
vegetable that grows
underground and is
good for eyesight.

(carrot)

---

2 points

True or false —
the healthiest person is the
one who doesn't eat *any* fat

(false — a small amount of fat is
an important part of the diet)

---

2 points

About how many calories
are in a Big Mac and
large order of fries —
200, 750, or 1,000?

(about 1,000 calories)

---

2 points

Name a high-fat
food that is found in a
vending machine.

(chips, chocolate bar, cookies . . .)

---

2 points

Name two foods that
begin with "C" that are
very high in sugar.

(cookies, cake, candy, cola)

---

2 points

How much sugar is in one
regular can of Coke —
*2 teaspoons, 5 teaspoons, or
10 teaspoons?*

(10 teaspoons of sugar)

---

2 points

Name a high-fat liquid that
is sometimes served over
mashed potatoes.

(gravy, melted butter)

---

2 points

How many chips make up one
serving of potato chips —
about . . . 2 chips, 14 chips, or 25 chips?

(about 14 chips)

2 points

Name a fruit that grows on a vine

(grapes, pumpkin)

2 points

Name a vegetable that may have a purple color

(eggplant, beet)

2 points

Name the main ingredient in white bread.

(flour)

2 points

Name a high fat food that is served on top of pancakes

(butter)

2 points

Name a vegetable (often found in salad) that has a shape like a banana

(cucumber)

2 points

Name a fruit that has a pit in its center

(cherry, peach, plum, date)

1 point

1 point

1 point

1 point

1 point

1 point

1 point

1 point

Gamesheet

4

2 points	2 points
2 points	2 points
2 points	2 points
2 points	2 points

Nutrition and Physical Activity Physical Education Lessons and Micro-Units

part IV

Physical Education Lessons

The physical education setting provides an ideal opportunity to teach students about the importance of both regular physical activity *and* good nutrition. Complementing the themes of the classroom lessons included in parts I and II, the physical education lessons in part IV incorporate key nutrition concepts into physical education class. Designed to be taught by a school's physical education teacher, these lessons are based on the five-part framework of the safe workout. Each physical activity lesson actually leads students through the five steps:

1. Warm-up
2. Stretch
3. Fitness activity—an active game that involves a nutrition concept
4. Cool-down
5. Cool-down stretch

In addition to emphasizing the five parts to a safe workout as well as incorporating key nutritional concepts, these lessons also focus on endurance fitness activities. Depending on the fitness levels of your students, you may want to modify these activities and slowly build up to and even beyond the target levels.

Three Kinds of Fitness Fun: Endurance, Strength, and Flexibility

Background

Fitness consists of three components—endurance, strength, and flexibility. Students should understand that each of these is important and needs to be addressed in order for students to become totally fit.

Each component of fitness has an important job for the body. **Endurance fitness** helps with heart health and weight maintenance. The key to endurance fitness is to exercise for an extended period of time without stopping. Choosing an appropriate pace is very important when doing an endurance activity. Students should not exert themselves so hard that they get tired after only a few minutes. Regular training is also important in developing endurance fitness. Students should do an aerobic activity at least three times per week. Examples of endurance workouts are jumping rope, cycling, walking, jogging, dancing, and any other activity that is performed continuously.

To develop **strength fitness**, one must perform exercises that make muscles work harder than they are used to. This is called overloading. The muscles must be challenged to go farther, to lift something heavier, or to go faster than they usually do. The muscle fibers that make up muscles get thicker and stronger when they are overloaded regularly. Examples of exercises that improve strength fitness include sit-ups, crunches, push-ups, weight-lifting, and climbing. Sports in which strength fitness is important include basketball, baseball, tennis, and track and field.

Flexibility fitness is important because it helps prevent injuries and helps the body move more efficiently. The way you improve flexibility fitness is by stretching. Stretching on a regular basis will improve the range of motion of the joints and lengthen the fibers of muscles so they will move better with fewer chances of injury. Stretching should be done slowly and properly. Holding a stretch for ten seconds or more helps muscles become more flexible. Flexibility fitness is very important in all sports.

It is extremely important for students to practice what they learn in physical education class and make fitness part of their lifestyle at home as well.

Estimated Teaching Time

Estimated teaching time: 30 minutes

Objectives

1. The students will demonstrate the five parts of the safe workout.
2. The students will demonstrate different exercises that help improve endurance, strength, and flexibility fitness.
3. The students will be able to identify the different parts of fitness and which exercises improve specific areas of fitness.

Materials

1. Fitness cards: cards listing an exercise (e.g., push-ups)
2. Fifteen containers (e.g., paper grocery bags)
3. Examples of stretches and strength fitness activities (see appendix pp. 453-459)

Safety Points

1. Keep movements fluid and in control.
2. Perform exercises with the proper form.
3. Perform the five parts of the safe workout properly.

Procedure

1. Have students form five groups. (The number of students in a group will depend on the class size; you could have more or less than five groups.)
2. Place fitness cards face up on the side of gym opposite students (see figure 29.1). Cards may have to be duplicated more than once so that there are enough for each student to have a turn.

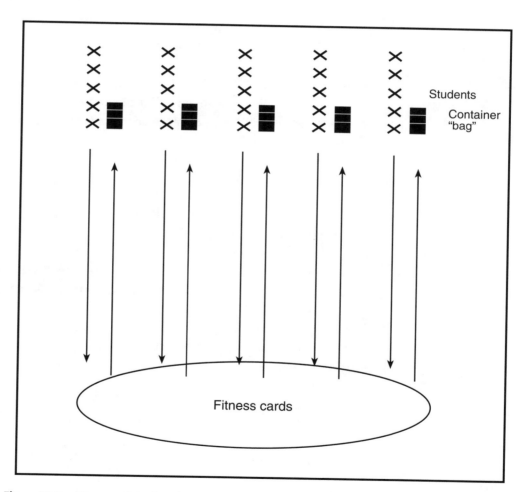

Figure 29.1 Fitness activity line formation.

3. Place three containers next to each group. One container will be used for each area of fitness. These will be used to collect the fitness cards chosen by each group.

4. Lead the students in a warm-up and stretch. Review with students the important points of a warm-up and stretch as well as the importance of endurance and strength fitness activities.

a. Warm-up

1) Benefits of warming up

- Helps prevent injuries.
- Increases body temperature.
- Gets the body ready for the rest of the workout.

2) How to warm up

- Perform a series of slow movements for 5-10 minutes.
- Examples include slow jogging in place, slow jumping jacks.

b. Stretch

1) Benefits of stretching

- Improves flexibility fitness.
- Improves the ability of muscles to work.
- Improves the body's ability to move.
- Decreases the number of injuries.

2) How to stretch (see appendix for diagrams, pp. 453-456)

- Hold stretch for 10 or more seconds (count out loud: 1 Mississippi, 2 Mississippi . . . to 10 Mississippi).
- Don't bounce, hold stretch gently.
- Stretch slowly.
- Use proper form to avoid injuries.
- Examples: neck stretch, butterfly, quad burner (thigh stretch).

c. Strength fitness (see appendix for diagrams, pp. 457-459)

1) Benefits of strength fitness

- Improves the ability of your muscles to move or resist a force or workload.
- Helps you perform your daily tasks without getting tired.
- Helps prevent injuries.
- Improves your skills in games and sports—e.g., jumping rope, playing dodge ball, shooting a basketball.

2) How to improve strength fitness

- Make your muscles work more than they are used to—e.g., go faster, go longer, lift heavier objects, exercise more often.
- Train, don't strain.
- Not too much, too soon, or too often.

d. Endurance fitness

1) Benefits of endurance fitness

- Helps improve heart, lungs, and blood-vessel health (cardiovascular fitness).
- Helps maintain a healthy weight.
- Gives you energy.

2) How to improve endurance fitness

- Do nonstop, continuous movement activities—e.g., nonstop bike riding, nonstop walking, nonstop rope jumping (students may jog or walk in place to demonstrate endurance activities in class).
- Find a pace (speed) you can do for a long time—"Pace, don't race!"
- As a goal, do endurance activities three to four days a week for 20-30 minutes.
- Find an endurance activity you like so you will want to do it.

5. Explain to the students that they will be performing an endurance fitness activity so they need to find a pace, or "speed," that they can do for a long time without stopping. Remind students to "Pace, don't race!" Stress that the speed they pick needs to be a pace that works for them, and that they shouldn't worry about how other students are doing.

6. Explain that at the other end of the gym there are fitness cards with exercises listed on them. Each exercise addresses a different area of fitness. Review the three different parts of fitness with students. Talk about exercises that would improve endurance fitness, strength fitness, and flexibility fitness.

7. On your signal, have the first person in each line jog/run to the fitness cards and pick one up. The first one they touch is the one they bring back to the group.

8. When they get back to the group, they should place the fitness card into the container representing the area of fitness the card addresses. The student should then go to the end of the line. Remember, everyone should be pacing during the entire time! When waiting in line, students should be marching or jogging in place.

9. Keep this going until: (a) the fitness cards are gone, (b) each student has gone a designated number of times, or (c) time becomes a concern.

10. Have the groups then review their choices, making sure all cards are correctly classified.

11. Have each group share its choices with the class. Correct any incorrectly classified fitness cards.

12. Have each group demonstrate a fitness activity that they feel would work well at home. Make sure that each area of fitness is covered at least once.

13. Repeat fitness activity if time allows.

14. Lead students in a cool-down and cool-down stretch. Review the important points of each with them.

    a. Cool-down

      1) Benefits of cooling down
- Lets the body slow down or recover from the fitness activity.
- Helps prevent injuries and muscle soreness.

      2) How to cool down
- Walk slowly.
- Walk in place slowly.

    b. Cool-down stretch (see the appendix)

      1) Benefits of the cool-down stretch
- Helps prevent soreness.
- Improves flexibility fitness.

      2) How to do the cool-down stretch
- Hold stretch for 10 or more seconds (count out loud: 1 Mississippi, 2 Mississippi . . . to 10 Mississippi).
- Examples: neck stretch, butterfly, quad burner (thigh stretch).

Overview of fitness cards

Endurance fitness	Strength fitness	Flexibility fitness
Swimming	Push-ups	Neck stretch
Jumping rope	Sit-ups	Arm stretch
Power walking	Weight lifting	Palms to ceiling
Dancing	Pull-ups	Reach back
Basketball	Crunches	Hold up the wall
Jogging	Climbing	Shoulder stretch
In-line skating	Chin-ups	The wave
Ice hockey	Wall sits	Quad burner
Cycling		Butterfly
Running		Hamstring stretch

swimming	jogging
jumping rope	in-line skating
power walking	ice hockey
dancing	cycling

basketball	running
push-ups	crunches
sit-ups	climbing
weight lifting	chin-ups

pull-ups	butterfly
neck stretch	shoulder stretch
palms to ceiling	quad burner
reach back	hamstring stretch

hold up the wall	the wave
arm stretch	

Five Foods Countdown

Background

The combination of a healthy diet and physical activity is important to good health. This message has been emphasized in the fourth and fifth grade classroom lessons, and this physical education lesson provides an opportunity to further reinforce this message with students.

In this lesson, students will review nutritional concepts while simultaneously moving around the gymnasium. The lesson will help to reinforce knowledge of nutrition, and provide an opportunity for students to enhance their motor skills through physical activity.

The gymnasium is a perfect classroom in which to learn. Students should understand that Physical Education is a class for learning, and they need to enter the gym knowing that although there are no desks, chairs, or pencils, they will be learning important information. Because children love to move, this lesson provides an opportunity for students not only to improve their fitness but also to have fun while learning about issues important to their lifelong health.

This lesson takes approximately thirty minutes to complete and leads students through the five parts of the safe workout, while also reviewing the food groups of the Food Guide Pyramid.

Estimated Teaching Time

Estimated teaching time: 30 minutes

Objectives

1. The students will be able to complete an endurance workout.
2. The students will demonstrate a pace that works for them so that they can move for a long time without stopping.
3. The students will be able to list a variety of foods from the food groups of the Food Guide Pyramid.

Materials

1. Music (medium/up-tempo)
2. Teacher Resource Page #1

Safety Points

1. Move with control throughout the activity
2. Pace yourself so you have enough energy to do safe movements throughout the activity

Procedure

1. Assemble students in an appropriate formation that allows them room to move (circle or scattered formation); then lead them through a warm-up and stretch, while reviewing the important points of warming up and stretching.

   a. Warm-up

      1) Benefits of warming up

         - Helps prevent injuries.
         - Increases body temperature.
         - Gets the body ready for the rest of the workout.

      2) How to warm up

         - Perform a series of slow movements for 5-10 minutes.
         - Examples include slow jogging in place, slow jumping jacks.

   b. Stretch

      1) Benefits of stretching

         - Improves flexibility fitness.
         - Improves the ability of muscles to work.
         - Improves the body's ability to move.
         - Decreases the number of injuries.

      2) How to stretch (see the appendix, pp. 453-456)

         - Hold stretch for 10 or more seconds (count out loud: 1 Mississippi, 2 Mississippi . . . to 10 Mississippi).
         - Don't bounce, hold stretch gently.
         - Stretch slowly.
         - Use proper form to avoid injuries.
         - Examples: neck stretch, butterfly, quad burner (thigh stretch).

2. As students are moving and stretching, review with them the important aspects of endurance and strength fitness activities.

   a. Strength fitness (see the appendix, pp. 457-459)

      1) Benefits of strength fitness

         - Improves the ability of your muscles to move or resist a force or workload.
         - Helps you perform your daily tasks without getting tired.
         - Helps prevent injuries.
         - Improves your skills in games and sports—e.g., jumping rope, playing dodge ball, shooting a basketball.

      2) How to improve strength fitness

         - Make your muscles work more than they are used to—e.g., go faster, go longer, lift heavier objects, exercise more often.
         - Train, don't strain.
         - Not too much, too soon, or too often.

b. Endurance fitness
   1) Benefits of endurance fitness
      • Helps improve heart, lungs, and blood-vessel health (cardiovascular fitness).
      • Helps maintain a healthy weight.
      • Gives you energy.
   2) How to improve endurance fitness
      • Do nonstop, continuous movement activities—e.g., nonstop bike riding, nonstop walking, nonstop rope jumping (students may jog or walk in place to demonstrate endurance activities in class).
      • Find a pace (speed) you can do for a long time—"Pace, don't race!"
      • As a goal, do endurance activities three to four days a week for 20-30 minutes.
      • Find an endurance activity you like so you will want to do it.
3. After the warm-up and stretch, have students practice jogging or walking at an endurance pace (a pace they can do for a long time) as they move in the same direction around the perimeter of the gym (see figure 30.1).

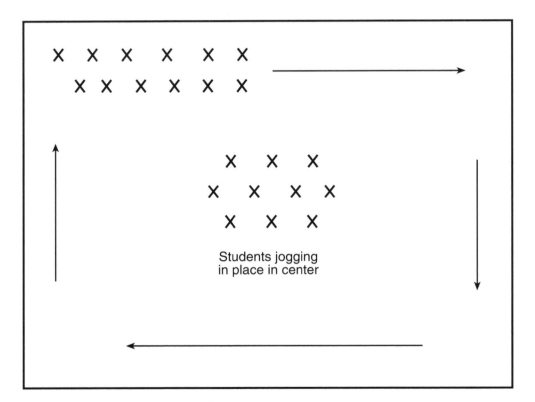

X = Students

Figure 30.1   Fitness activity line formation.

4. Stress to students the importance of finding their own pace—a pace that works for them (not a friend) and a speed they can do without getting tired.
5. Pick two students to demonstrate the "Five Foods Countdown" activity.

6. Have students face each other and put one hand out in front of them, in a fist at waist level.

7. Then announce a food group, e.g., fruit group. The two students take turns naming foods from the fruit group. As they announce each food, they extend a finger on their hand while making the arm motion of an umpire calling a strike. With each food they name, they extend another finger, until all five fingers are extended. For example, one student says "apple" as he/she makes the arm motion and extends a finger, then the other student says "pear" and does the same. (Other counting motions may be used as well. For example, students could pat hands, shake hands, slap hands, or even do some kind of movements with their feet.)

8. After the demonstration of the "Five Foods Countdown" activity, have the other students practice with each other.

9. When the class is ready, start the music, and have the children start moving (walking/jogging, for example) in the same direction around the perimeter of the gym. After each round of Five Foods Countdown, students can reverse direction. Those students who want to jog/walk in place during the activity can do so in the center of the gym. (See figure 30.1)

10. Stress pacing to students and have them use a variety of locomotive skills throughout the activity—e.g., walking, jogging, skipping, etc. You can specify the movements, or leave the choice to your students.

11. While the students move around the gym, stop the music and announce a food group. The students need to find the closest partner and start counting out five foods that come from the announced food group. Remind students to make sure their partner is only naming foods that belong in the announced food group. Students must work with a different partner each time a food group is called.

12. Besides food groups, you can also have students name low-fat breakfast foods, snack foods, lunch foods, etc.

13. When the class gets enough experience and endurance with the activity, the students can keep moving (jogging in place, for example) while they count their five foods.

14. Lead students in a cool-down and cool-down stretch. Review the important points of each with them. Likewise, review the foods or food groups they had difficulty with during the activity.

    a. Cool-down

       1) Benefits of cooling down

          - Lets the body slow down or recover from the fitness activity.
          - Helps prevent injuries and muscle soreness.

       2) How to cool down

          - Walk slowly.
          - Walk in place slowly.

    b. Cool-down stretch

       1) Benefits of the cool-down stretch

          - Helps prevent soreness.
          - Improves flexibility fitness.

       2) How to do the cool-down stretch

          - Hold stretch for 10 or more seconds (count out loud: 1 Mississippi, 2 Mississippi . . . to 10 Mississippi).
          - Examples: neck stretch, butterfly, quad burner (thigh stretch).

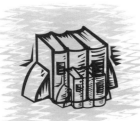

Teacher Resource Page #1

Over the years, experts have formed guidelines to help Americans eat better in order to keep us healthier and to enhance our quality of life. The Food Guide Pyramid—a concept developed by the United States Department of Agriculture (USDA)—represents years of research on what a healthy diet is for Americans over two years of age.

This research focused on what foods Americans eat now, what nutrients are in the foods we eat, and how these patterns need to change to better prevent disease and promote good health. The Food Guide Pyramid promotes moderation, variety, and balance. The pyramid will help you choose what and how much to eat from each food group to get the nutrients you need, without getting too many calories, too much fat, saturated fat, cholesterol, sugar, sodium, or alcohol.

There are six categories in the pyramid, and the size of each category corresponds to the amount of food from that group that you need to eat each day. The groups toward the bottom of the pyramid take up more space, which means that you need more of these foods and less of the foods closer to the top. The food group at the tip of the pyramid is for fat and sugar. It is healthy to eat these only in small amounts. For instance, a low-fat diet may help your body avoid heart disease and some types of cancer, as well as help your body maintain a healthy weight.

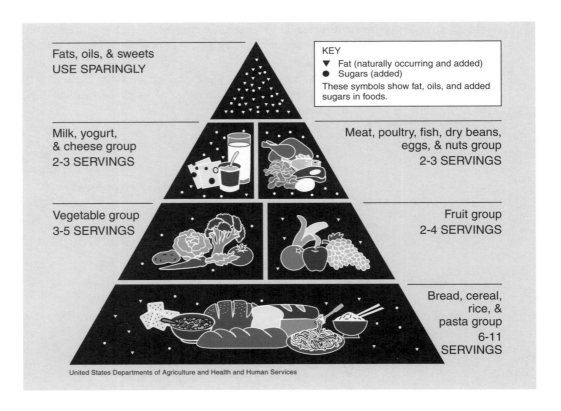

Fats, oils, & sweets
USE SPARINGLY

KEY
▼ Fat (naturally occurring and added)
● Sugars (added)
These symbols show fat, oils, and added sugars in foods.

Milk, yogurt,
& cheese group
2-3 SERVINGS

Meat, poultry, fish, dry beans,
eggs, & nuts group
2-3 SERVINGS

Vegetable group
3-5 SERVINGS

Fruit group
2-4 SERVINGS

Bread, cereal,
rice, &
pasta group
6-11
SERVINGS

United States Departments of Agriculture and Health and Human Services

Examples of Food Items That Belong in Each Food Group

Food Group	Food Items
Grain (bread, cereal, rice, and pasta)	Whole grain bread, corn bread, muffins, rolls, wheat bread, biscuits, pancakes, pretzels, cereal, rice, and pasta (macaroni, spaghetti)
Vegetable	Collard greens, mustard greens, spinach, kale, corn, turnips, lima beans, string beans, cabbage, white potatoes, sweet potatoes, broccoli, carrots, okra, squash
Fruit	Peaches, nectarines, cantaloupe, watermelon, grapefruit, raisins, apples, oranges, bananas, strawberries
Meat, poultry, fish, dry beans, eggs, and nuts	Peanut butter, kidney beans, navy beans, black-eyed peas, peanuts, lean-cut meat, chicken, turkey, beef, fish, eggs
Dairy (milk, yogurt, and cheese)	Nonfat milk, 1% milk, 2% milk, cottage cheese, cheddar cheese, American cheese, frozen yogurt

Musical Fare

Background

The combination of a healthy diet and physical activity is important to good health. This message has been emphasized in the fourth and fifth grade classroom lessons, and this physical education lesson provides an opportunity to further reinforce this message with students.

In this lesson, students will review nutritional concepts while simultaneously moving around the gymnasium. The lesson will help to reinforce nutritional knowledge, as well as provide an opportunity for students to enhance their motor skills through physical activity.

The gymnasium is a perfect classroom in which to learn. Students should understand that Physical Education is a class for learning, and they need to enter the gym knowing that although there are no desks, chairs, or pencils, they will be learning important information as they are moving. Because children love to move, this lesson provides an opportunity for students not only to improve their fitness but also to have fun while learning about issues important to their lifelong health.

This lesson takes approximately thirty minutes to complete and leads students through a warm-up and stretch; a fitness activity game similar to musical chairs but using food pictures; and finally, a cool-down and cool-down stretch.

Estimated Teaching Time

Estimated teaching time: 30 minutes

Objectives

1. Students will demonstrate an endurance workout while pacing themselves during the fitness activity.
2. Students will demonstrate a pace that works for them so that they can move for a long time without stopping.
3. Students will demonstrate their knowledge of the Food Guide Pyramid's food groups and recommended servings per day.

Materials

1. Music (medium/up-tempo)
2. Food pictures (cut out from magazines, food packages, or available from many state dairy councils)
3. Teacher Resource Page #1

Safety Points

1. Move with control throughout the exercise.
2. Pace yourself to allow safe, fluid movements throughout the lesson.
3. Move around the food pictures without stepping or slipping on them.

Procedure

1. Assemble students in an appropriate formation (circle or scattered formation) and lead them through a warm-up and stretch, while reviewing important points of the warm-up and stretch.
   a. Warm-up
      1) Benefits of warming up
         - Helps prevent injuries.
         - Increases body temperature.
         - Gets the body ready for the rest of the workout.
      2) How to warm up
         - Perform a series of slow movements for 5-10 minutes.
         - Examples include slow jogging in place, slow jumping jacks.
   b. Stretch
      1) Benefits of stretching
         - Improves flexibility fitness.
         - Improves the ability of muscles to work.
         - Improves the body's ability to move.
         - Decreases the number of injuries.
      2) How to stretch (see the appendix, pp. 453-456)
         - Hold stretch for 10 or more seconds (count out loud: 1 Mississippi, 2 Mississippi . . . to 10 Mississippi).
         - Don't bounce, hold stretch gently.
         - Stretch slowly.
         - Use proper form to avoid injuries.
         - Examples: neck stretch, butterfly, quad burner (thigh stretch).
2. Review with students the important aspects of endurance and strength fitness activities.
   a. Strength fitness (see the appendix, pp. 457-459)
      1) Benefits of strength fitness
         - Improves the ability of your muscles to move or resist a force or workload.
         - Helps you perform your daily tasks without getting tired.
         - Helps prevent injuries.
         - Improves your skills in games and sports—e.g., jumping rope, playing dodge ball, shooting a basketball.
      2) How to improve strength fitness
         - Make your muscles work more than they are used to—e.g., go faster, go longer, lift heavier objects, exercise more often.
         - Train, don't strain.
         - Not too much, too soon, or too often.
   b. Endurance fitness
      1) Benefits of endurance fitness
         - Helps improve heart, lungs, and blood-vessel health (cardiovascular fitness).

- Helps maintain a healthy weight.
- Gives you energy.

2) How to improve endurance fitness
- Do nonstop, continuous movement activities—e.g., nonstop bike riding, nonstop walking, nonstop rope jumping (students may jog or walk in place to demonstrate endurance activities in class).
- Find a pace (speed) you can do for a long time—"Pace, don't race!"
- As a goal, do endurance activities three to four days a week for 20-30 minutes.
- Find an endurance activity you like so you will want to do it.

3. Have the students find their own space in the gym and practice moving (e.g., jogging in place) at an endurance pace (a pace they can do for a long time).

4. Stress the importance of finding their own pace, a pace that works for them, not a friend, but a speed they can do without getting tired.

5. Place food pictures from all the food groups around the perimeter of the gym and up against the wall (see figure 31.1). Make sure the pictures are not too close to one another.

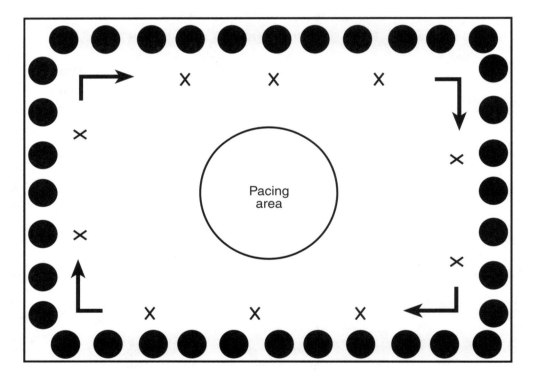

● = Food pictures

X = Students

Figure 31.1 Fitness activity formation.

6. Explain to students that the pictures come from all five of the "all of the time" food groups of the Food Guide Pyramid.

7. Ask them what group that people should use sparingly is missing (the fats, oils, and sweets group).

8. Review with students the different food groups as well as recommended servings per day from the different groups. (While doing this, you can have students place the food pictures around the gym).

9. Have music ready to go. (Music must be able to be turned on and off easily.)

10. Explain to students that they will be playing an endurance game that is like musical chairs—but using food pictures rather than chairs.

11. Stress that students will be active throughout the workout and that pacing themselves is important, so that they will not get tired. They should find a speed (pace) that they can do for a long time.

12. Explain to students that they may use a different locomotive skill for each round of the game. One round they could jog; one round they could walk; one round they could skip; etc.

13. When the music begins, have students jog around the perimeter of the room (all in the same direction and spaced out appropriately) next to the food pictures. Remind students to be careful not to step on the pictures.

14. When the music stops, have each student stand next to the food picture he/she is closest to, pick it up, and hold it over his/her head. Then, you call out one or two food groups (the number of food groups you call out will depend on the class size). Those students who do not have a food that belongs to the announced food groups put their pictures down where they found them and go to an area of the room called the "pacing" area, where they will remain (and continue walking or jogging in place) for one round.

15. Have students double-check with their neighbors to make sure they have correctly determined if their food does or does not belong to the announced food group. You can make the final determination if students are unclear on the correct answer.

16. Have students in the pacing area return to the main group, after having missed one round (where a new food group is called).

Sample Round

When the music stops, each student picks up the food picture he/she is closest to and holds it above his/her head. Then you call out "grain group" and "dairy group." Students check their foods with their neighbors, and those students who do not have a food picture belonging to the grain or dairy group put their pictures down and go to the pacing area. The rest of the students then put their pictures back down on the ground, and you start the music again to begin another round.

17. Lead students in a cool-down and cool-down stretch. Review the important points of each with them.
    a. Cool-down
       1) Benefits of cooling down
          • Lets the body slow down or recover from the fitness activity.
          • Helps prevent injuries and muscle soreness.

2) How to cool down
- Walk slowly.
- Walk in place slowly.

b. Cool-down stretch

1) Benefits of the cool-down stretch
- Helps prevent soreness.
- Improves flexibility fitness.

2) How to do the cool-down stretch
- Hold stretch for 10 or more seconds (count out loud: 1 Mississippi, 2 Mississippi . . . to 10 Mississippi).
- Examples: neck stretch, butterfly, quad burner (thigh stretch).

Teacher Resource Page #1

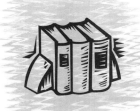

Using the Game to Teach Recommended Servings Per Day

After students master the activity, you may introduce into the game the concept of recommended servings per day.

1. After the students find the food pictures of the food group, ask a student to choose the correct servings per day of that group by picking, for example, 6-11 favorite foods from the grain group choices.

2. Each time the music stops, another student can select his/her favorite choices to meet the recommended daily servings. The student who chooses the daily servings can be the "teacher" and turn the music on, and call out the next food group. Depending on the class size and number of pictures, more than one student can pick the servings per day of the food group.

Additional Game Variations

In order to keep the game exciting, you may want to modify it every once in awhile.

1. Have students pair up and work as partners to play the game.

2. Change the rules so those who have pictures of the food group called move into the pacing area.

Food Guide Pyramid

Over the years, experts have formed guidelines to help Americans eat better in order to keep us healthier and to enhance our quality of life. The Food Guide Pyramid—a concept developed by the United States Department of Agriculture (USDA)—represents years of research on what a healthy diet is for Americans over two years of age.

This research focused on what foods Americans eat now, what nutrients are in the foods we eat, and how these patterns need to change to better prevent disease and promote good health. The Food Guide Pyramid promotes moderation, variety, and balance. The pyramid will help you choose what and how much to eat from each food group to get the nutrients you need, without getting too many calories, too much fat, saturated fat, cholesterol, sugar, sodium, or alcohol.

There are six categories in the pyramid, and the size of each category corresponds to the amount of food from that group that you need to eat each day. The groups toward the bottom of the pyramid take up more space, which means that you need more of these foods and less of the foods closer to the top. The food group at the tip of the pyramid is for fat and sugar. It is healthy to eat these only in small amounts. For instance, a low-fat diet may help your body avoid heart disease and some types of cancer, as well as help your body maintain a healthy weight.

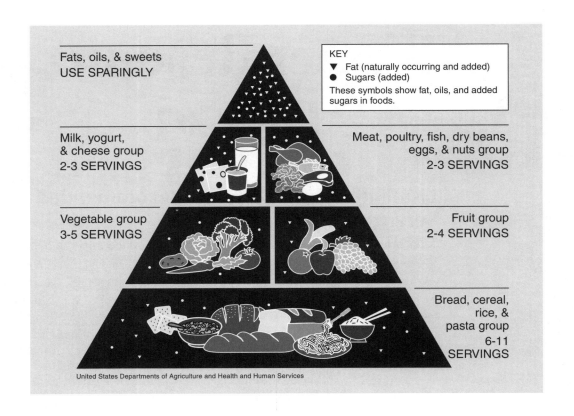

Fats, oils, & sweets
USE SPARINGLY

KEY
▼ Fat (naturally occurring and added)
● Sugars (added)
These symbols show fat, oils, and added sugars in foods.

Milk, yogurt,
& cheese group
2-3 SERVINGS

Meat, poultry, fish, dry beans,
eggs, & nuts group
2-3 SERVINGS

Vegetable group
3-5 SERVINGS

Fruit group
2-4 SERVINGS

Bread, cereal,
rice, &
pasta group
6-11
SERVINGS

United States Departments of Agriculture and Health and Human Services

Examples of Food Items That Belong in Each Food Group

Food Group	Food Items
Grain (bread, cereal, rice, and pasta)	Whole grain bread, corn bread, muffins, rolls, wheat bread, biscuits, pancakes, pretzels, cereal, rice, and pasta (macaroni, spaghetti)
Vegetable	Collard greens, mustard greens, spinach, kale, corn, turnips, lima beans, string beans, cabbage, white potatoes, sweet potatoes, broccoli, carrots, okra, squash
Fruit	Peaches, nectarines, cantaloupe, watermelon, grapefruit, raisins, apples, oranges, bananas, strawberries
Meat, poultry, fish, dry beans, eggs, and nuts	Peanut butter, kidney beans, navy beans, black-eyed peas, peanuts, lean-cut meat, chicken, turkey, beef, fish, eggs
Dairy (milk, yogurt, and cheese)	Nonfat milk, 1% milk, 2% milk, cottage cheese, cheddar cheese, American cheese, frozen yogurt

Bowling for Snacks

Background

This lesson will help students understand how important physical activity and eating healthful snacks are for a healthy body.

Snacks can be an important part of a child's diet. Healthful snacks can help provide the calories and nutrients children need for growth and development. Children need guidance, however. They often choose snacks that are high in fat, sugar, salt, or calories and low in important nutrients such as vitamins and minerals. These types of snacks are said to be filled with "empty calories" because they provide many calories but few of the nutrients the body needs to stay healthy and grow strong.

Snacks such as fruit, low-fat yogurt, and whole wheat bread, on the other hand, are nutrient-dense, providing both calories and nutrients. Students need to understand the importance of choosing nutrient-dense snacks over snacks filled with empty calories.

In this lesson, students learn about choosing healthful, nutrient-dense snacks in a "bowling" activity. Cans representing healthful and less healthful snacks are set up in the gym and students attempt to knock over only those targets/pins representing healthful, nutrient-dense snacks.

Estimated Teaching Time

Estimated teaching time: 30 minutes

Objectives

1. The students will be able to complete an endurance workout.
2. The students will demonstrate a pace that they can follow for a long time without stopping.
3. The students will describe the difference between healthful, nutrient-dense snacks and "empty calorie" snacks.
4. The students will be able to categorize snacks into their appropriate food groups.

Materials

1. Approximately 30-50 pieces of equipment that will be used as targets/pins (such as tennis ball cans, milk cartons, soda cans, plastic soda bottles, Pringles cans, plastic cups, paper cups). Pictures of snacks will be attached to each target/pin.
2. Fifteen or more balls (e.g., yarn balls, Nerf balls, tennis balls, or any equipment that can be safely used to roll toward and knock down the target with the attached food picture).
3. A variety of nutrient-dense snack pictures and a variety of empty-calorie snack pictures (to be attached/taped to targets/pins). Students can bring in these pictures. They can cut them out of magazines and newspapers or bring in empty food packages. Classroom teachers may also have a collection of such pictures that could be used in this lesson.
4. Two sets of Food Guide Pyramid food group signs (one set of originals is provided).
5. Ten hula hoops (optional).
6. Teacher Resource Page #1

Safety Points

1. Choose equipment that is safe.
2. Provide enough open space for students to move freely without getting hurt.

Procedure

1. Lead students through a warm-up and stretch. Review the important points of warming up and stretching.
   a. Warm-up
      1) Benefits of warming up
         - Helps prevent injuries.
         - Increases body temperature.
         - Gets the body ready for the rest of the workout.
      2) How to warm up
         - Perform a series of slow movements for 5-10 minutes.
         - Examples include slow jogging in place, slow jumping jacks.
   b. Stretch
      1) Benefits of stretching
         - Improves flexibility fitness.
         - Improves the ability of muscles to work.
         - Improves the body's ability to move.
         - Decreases the number of injuries.
      2) How to stretch (see appendix, pp. 453-456)
         - Hold stretch for 10 or more seconds (count out loud: 1 Mississippi, 2 Mississippi . . . to 10 Mississippi).
         - Don't bounce, hold stretch gently.
         - Stretch slowly.
         - Use proper form to avoid injuries.
         - Examples: neck stretch, butterfly, quad burner (thigh stretch).
2. Review the important aspects of endurance fitness activities.
      1) Benefits of endurance fitness
         - Helps improve heart, lungs, and blood-vessel health (cardiovascular fitness).
         - Helps maintain a healthy weight.
         - Gives you energy.
      2) How to improve endurance fitness
         - Do nonstop, continuous movement activities—e.g., nonstop bike riding, nonstop walking, nonstop rope jumping (students may jog or walk in place to demonstrate endurance activities in class).
         - Find a pace (speed) you can do for a long time—"Pace, don't race!"
         - As a goal, do endurance activities three to four days a week for 20-30 minutes.
         - Find an endurance activity you like so you will want to do it.

3. Set up half of the cans with food pictures attached on one side of the gym and set up the other half on the other side of the gym (see figure 32.1). Make sure that healthful and less healthful snacks are distributed evenly throughout each side.

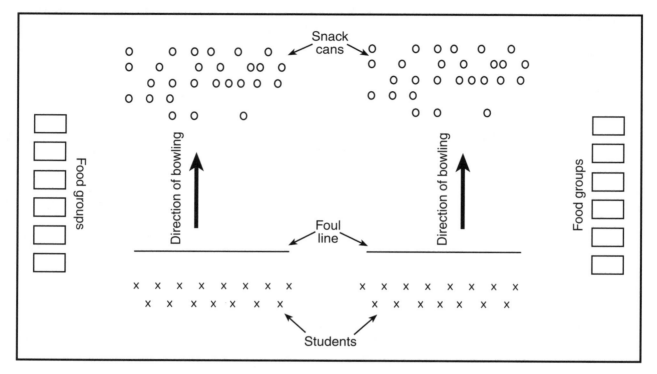

Figure 32.1 Fitness activity line formation.

4. If necessary, review with students the concept of bowling—rolling a ball down a lane to knock down pins.

5. Place the food group signs parallel to each team's bowling lane (see figure 32.1). If you want, place a hula hoop next to each food group sign. During the game, students can place their snack pictures in the proper hula hoops.

6. Review the rules of the game with students.

   a. How the game works: As in bowling, students use balls to knock over targets/pins. When a student is bowling, the objective is to knock over a target/pin that represents a healthful snack and then place this snack in its correct food group. The first team to knock down all its healthful snacks and have them correctly categorized into the different food groups wins the game.

   b. Game rules:

   - Students need to move nonstop for the entire game.
   - There will be two groups playing the game—one group on one side of the gym, the other on the other side (see figure 32.1).
   - Students may not cross the foul line when bowling (see figure 32.1).
   - Balls should be rolled underhand on the ground toward the targets/pins. They should not be thrown.
   - If the ball hits or knocks over a food-picture target/pin, the student may cross the foul line to see if the snack is a healthful snack or a less healthful snack.

- If it is a healthful snack, the student picks up the target and places it in the food group to which it belongs.
- If it is not a healthful snack, the student puts the target back, returns, then picks an exercise to complete (such as jumping jacks, push ups, sit ups, or pull ups) before getting to bowl again.
- The first group to knock down all their healthy snacks and place them in the correct food groups wins the game.
- The other team can send someone over to check to see that its opponent picked only healthy snacks and that the snacks were properly categorized.

7. After reviewing the rules, have students play the game.
8. Review the choices each group made when they were bowling and discuss the differences between healthful, nutrient-dense snacks (the ones they picked and placed in the food groups) and empty-calorie snacks (the ones that remain on the bowling lane).
9. Repeat game if time allows.
10. Lead students in a cool-down and cool-down stretch. Review the important points of each with them.
   a. Cool-down
      1) Benefits of cooling down
         - Lets the body slow down or recover from the fitness activity.
         - Helps prevent injuries and muscle soreness.
      2) How to cool down
         - Walk slowly.
         - Walk in place slowly.
   b. Cool-down stretch
      1) Benefits of the cool-down stretch
         - Helps prevent soreness.
         - Improves flexibility fitness.
      2) How to do the cool-down stretch
         - Hold stretch for 10 or more seconds (count out loud: 1 Mississippi, 2 Mississippi . . . to 10 Mississippi).
         - Examples: neck stretch, butterfly, quad burner (thigh stretch).

Teacher Resource Page #1

Variations of the Activity

You may want to change the activity to better fit your group needs, or to keep the activity fun and exciting.

1. Have the entire class work as one team. See how many healthful snacks the class can knock over and correctly classify in five minutes, and then see if they can beat their own score in the next five-minute round.

2. Have students switch from their dominant hand to non-dominant hand (or vice versa) with each new round.

Food Group Signs

One set of Food Guide Pyramid food group signs is included. However, be sure to make copies. You will want two copies of each sign for the activity.

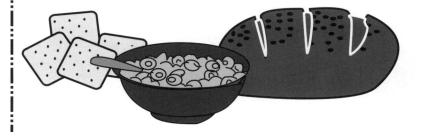

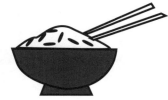

Grain

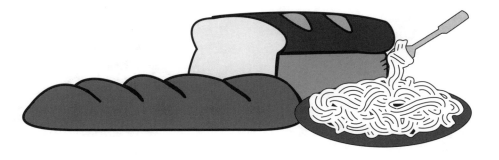

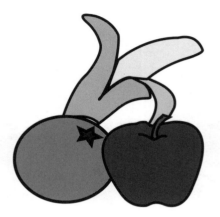

Fruit

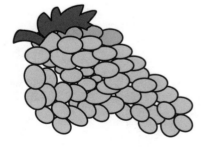

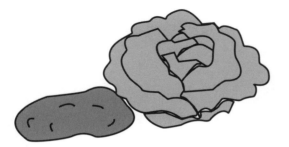

Vegetable

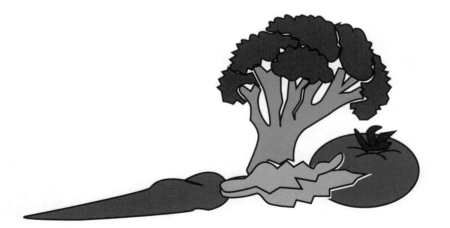

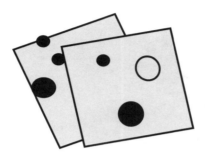

Dairy

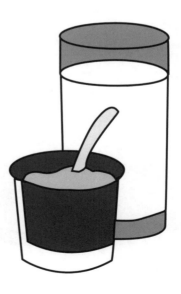

Meat, chicken, fish, and beans

Fruits and Vegetables

Background

Healthy bodies are the result of combining movement with eating right. This lesson stresses both. Students need to understand that exercising and eating right is a winning combination.

This lesson will help teach students the importance of choosing to eat at least five fruits and vegetables a day. Leading health authorities recommend that both adults and children eat at least five daily servings of fruits and vegetables. Getting 5-A-Day may help reduce the risk of cancer, obesity, diabetes, and heart disease. It's especially important to get children excited at a young age about getting 5-A-Day so that they establish healthy eating patterns that will last a lifetime.

This lesson takes approximately thirty minutes to complete and leads students through the five parts of a safe workout while also reviewing the fruits and vegetables groups of the Food Guide Pyramid.

Estimated Teaching Time

Estimated teaching time: 30 minutes

Objectives

1. The students will be able to complete an endurance workout.
2. The students will demonstrate a pace that works for them so that they can move for a long time without stopping.
3. The students will learn the importance of eating at least five servings of fruits and vegetables a day to help develop strong, healthy minds and bodies.

Materials

1. A large variety of food pictures showing (and/or food words naming) fruits, vegetables, and other food items. (There should be at least 45 fruits and vegetables.) Students can bring in these pictures. They can cut them out of magazines and newspapers or bring in empty food packages. Classroom teachers may also have a collection of such pictures that could be used in this lesson.

   Examples of fruits: apple, apricot, avocado, banana, cherry, coconut, date, fig, grape, grapefruit, kiwi, kumquat, lemon, lime, mango, melon, nectarine, orange, papaya, peach, pear, persimmon, pineapple, plum, prune, raisin, strawberry, tangerine

   Examples of vegetables: artichoke, asparagus, beet, broccoli, brussels sprouts, cabbage, carrot, cauliflower, celery, chard, corn, cucumber, eggplant, green beans, greens, kelp, lettuce, mushroom, okra, onion, parsnip, peas, pepper, pumpkin, radish, spinach, squash, sweet potato, tomato, turnip

   Examples of nonfruits/nonvegetables: barley, bread, butter, cashew, cheese, chicken, cookie, cracker, egg, tuna, tortilla, marshmallow, peanut, pork, salmon, shrimp, soda, wheat, yogurt

2. The phrase "5-A-Day" written on paper. (Each letter or number should be written on a separate piece of paper. For example, write the number "5" on one sheet of paper, the letter "A" on another, and so on. Each of the four teams will need a set of 5-A-Day sheets (see figure 33.1).

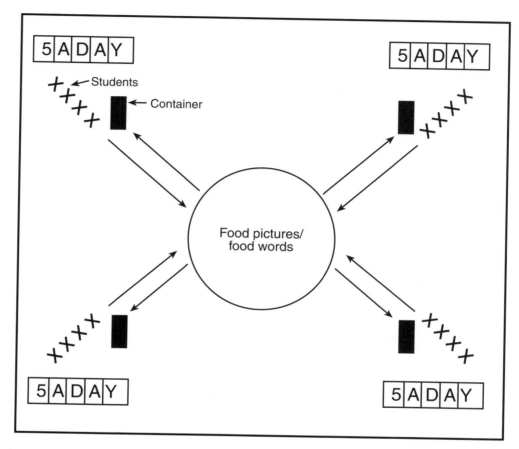

Figure 33.1 Fitness activity line formation.

3. Four containers (such as paper bags) in which each team can place the words or pictures of the items that are not fruits and vegetables (see figure 33.1).

Safety Points

1. Move with control throughout the exercise.
2. Pace yourself to allow safe, fluid movements throughout the lesson.

Procedure

1. Assemble students in an appropriate formation (circle or scattered formation) and lead them through a warm-up and stretch, while reviewing important points of a warm-up and stretch as well as the importance of endurance and strength fitness activities.

    a. Warm-up

      1) Benefits of warming up

- Helps prevent injuries.
- Increases body temperature.
- Gets the body ready for the rest of the workout.

      2) How to warm up

- Perform a series of slow movements for 5-10 minutes.
- Examples include slow jogging in place, slow jumping jacks.

    b. Stretch

      1) Benefits of stretching

- Improves flexibility fitness.
- Improves the ability of muscles to work.
- Improves the body's ability to move.
- Decreases the number of injuries.

      2) How to stretch (see appendix, pp. 453-456)

- Hold stretch for 10 or more seconds (count out loud: 1 Mississippi, 2 Mississippi . . . to 10 Mississippi).
- Don't bounce, hold stretch gently.
- Stretch slowly.
- Use proper form to avoid injuries.
- Examples: neck stretch, butterfly, quad burner (thigh stretch).

2. Review with students the important points of endurance and strength fitness activities.

    a. Strength fitness (see appendix, pp. 457-459)

      1) Benefits of strength fitness

- Improves the ability of your muscles to move or resist a force or workload.
- Helps you perform your daily tasks without getting tired.
- Helps prevent injuries.
- Improves your skills in games and sports—e.g., jumping rope, playing dodge ball, shooting a basketball.

      2) How to improve strength fitness

- Make your muscles work more than they are used to—e.g., go faster, go longer, lift heavier objects, exercise more often.
- Train, don't strain.
- Not too much, too soon, or too often.

    b. Endurance fitness

      1) Benefits of endurance fitness

- Helps improve heart, lungs, and blood-vessel health (cardiovascular fitness).
- Helps maintain a healthy weight.
- Gives you energy.

      2) How to improve endurance fitness

- Do nonstop, continuous movement activities—e.g., nonstop bike riding, nonstop walking, nonstop rope jumping (students may jog or walk in place to demonstrate endurance activities in class).

- Find a pace (speed) you can do for a long time—"Pace, don't race!"
- As a goal, do endurance activities three to four days a week for 20-30 minutes.
- Find an endurance activity you like so you will want to do it.

3. Divide students into four groups.

4. Place the food pictures and/or food words face down in the center of the room/gym (this can be done before or during class) and direct each group to move to a position equidistant from the pictures or food words.

5. Place a set of 5-A-Day letters next to each group, and have them lay out the sheets in an area where they will not get stepped on. Have the students stand near the container or bag, and line up one behind the other (see figure 33.1).

6. On your signal, the first person from each group should walk or jog (in control) to the food pictures/words, retrieve one, and then return to his/her group. (Note that the students picking up the picture or word card cannot peek at it until they return to their group. *Stress fair play.*)

   If the picture/word is a fruit or a vegetable, have the student put it on the first of the "5-A-Day" sheets—in this case, the paper that has the number "5." If the picture or food card is not a fruit or a vegetable, the student should put it in the container or bag.

   The next student should take a turn as soon as the first person gets back. The group is finished as soon as each sheet of paper used to spell "5-A-Day" is covered by a fruit or vegetable.

   Note: For a longer game, you can have students continue the game until all of the food pictures/words are gone. In this case, simply have the students keep filling in the letters of the "5-A-Day" sign, even if it means there is more than one picture on each letter.

7. Repeat the game by returning the food pictures/food words to the center of the gym and starting all over again.

   Remember: The students should be moving at a steady pace during the entire game! When they are waiting in line, they should be either marching or jogging in place.

8. For each round of the game, have each group review the fruits and vegetables covering their 5-A-Day sign.

9. Ask students why it is they should always get at least five servings of fruits and vegetables every day. Possible answers: it will give them energy; it will help them grow; it will keep them healthy.

10. Lead students in a cool-down and cool-down stretch. Review the important points of each with them.
    a. Cool-down
       1) Benefits of cooling down
          - Lets the body slow down or recover from the fitness activity.
          - Helps prevent injuries and muscle soreness.
       2) How to cool down
          - Walk slowly.
          - Walk in place slowly.

b. Cool-down stretch
 1) Benefits of the cool-down stretch
    - Helps prevent soreness.
    - Improves flexibility fitness.
 2) How to do the cool-down stretch
    - Hold stretch for 10 or more seconds (count out loud: 1 Mississippi, 2 Mississippi . . . to 10 Mississippi).
    - Examples: neck stretch, butterfly, quad burner (thigh stretch).

apples	apricots
avocados	bananas
strawberries	cherries
blueberries	raspberries
blackberries	boysenberries

coconuts	dates
figs	grapes
grapefruit	kiwi
kumquats	lemons
limes	mangoes

melons	nectarines
oranges	papayas
peaches	pears
persimmons	pineapples
plums	prunes

raisins	tangerines

artichokes	asparagus
beets	broccoli
brussels sprouts	carrots
cabbage	celery
cauliflower	corn

Swiss chard	eggplant
cucumbers	collard greens
green beans	iceberg lettuce
kelp	okra
mushrooms	parsnips

onions	peppers
peas	radishes
pumpkin	squash
spinach	tomatoes
sweet potatoes	turnips

dandelion greens	tofu
romaine lettuce	arugula
green leaf lettuce	dried beans
red leaf lettuce	legumes

flour tortillas	peanuts
cashews	cookies
yogurt	butter
eggs	cheese
chicken	soda

crackers	bread
salmon	bass
shrimp	pork
wheat	barley
marshmallows	

FitCheck
Guide

Part V includes both the Teachers' Guide to the FitCheck and the Students' Guide to the FitCheck. These resources were adapted from the middle-school curriculum, Planet Health*, and they are designed to teach teachers and students how to evaluate fitness progress

* Planet Health: Jill Carter, Jean Wiecha, Karen E. Peterson, and Steven L. Gortmaker, Human Kinetics, 2000.

Teachers' Guide to the FitCheck

FitCheck Overview

The FitCheck is a self-assessment tool that physical educators can use to help children identify, understand, and reflect upon their own patterns of physical activity and inactivity. Use it if it matches your students' abilities and fits into your curriculum. This version is simplified from *Planet Health,* which targets middle-school students.

FitCheck Components

1. *Planet Health* FitCheck journal (see pp. 406-407): Students fill this out at home over a seven-day period and translate their results into FitScores and SitScores.
2. Goal Setting Sheet (see p. 408): Students set goals based on their FitScores and SitScores.
3. FitScore and SitScore Progress Charts (see p. 409 and 410): Students record their scores on this chart when they complete each FitCheck or at two or three times you select during the year (try to make one time close to the end of the school year).

Using the FitCheck Journal

Lessons 35 through 39 introduce the FitCheck to students:

- *Lesson 35, Students' Guide to the FitCheck.*
- *Lesson 36, Charting Your FitScore and SitScore:* This lesson introduces the FitCheck journal.
- *Lesson 37, What Could You Do Instead of Watching TV?:* This is one of two lessons preparing students for goal setting (Lesson 39). It presents recommendations for limiting TV use and offers alternatives to television, video and computer games, and video tapes and movies.
- *Lesson 38, Making Time to Stay Fit:* This is the second lesson preparing students for goal setting (Lesson 39). Students make a group goal for class that day and evaluate their progress at the end of class. You may want to do this lesson several times with students until they are comfortable with goal setting and evaluation.
- *Lesson 39, Setting Goals for Personal Fitness:* Students set goals to improve their SitScore and FitScore. At the next FitCheck they evaluate their progress.

Using the FitScore and SitScore Progress Charts

There is no micro-unit to accompany the progress charts (see p. 409 and 410). After completing each FitCheck, or at two to three times during the school year, teachers should have students graph their scores so they can see how their progress over time. This is an activity that could be coordinated with a math teacher, or even carried out in math class.

Tips for Teaching the FitCheck

1. Read through all the FitCheck units (36 through 39) first.
2. Plan a schedule of FitChecks for the year. We recommend doing one two to three times during the school year. You can spread out journal assignments, charting,

and goal setting/goal evaluation over several classes to maximize physical activity time in your classes. If your students are not able to handle goal setting and evaluation, you can still do the journals.

3. Set up a filing system.

4. Coordinate with other teachers.

   - Because FitChecks require homework, you may want to coordinate with your students' classroom teachers ahead of time.

   - You may want to coordinate with a math teacher to do the bar graph exercise (FitScore and SitScore Progress Chart; see pp. 409 and 410).

5. Help students compare their FitScores and SitScores to expert recommendations for children.

   - The National Association for Sport and Physical Activity (NASPE 1998) recommends that "elementary school-age children should accumulate at least 30-60 minutes of activity from a variety of activities on all or most days of the week." Up to several hours per day is fine, too. NASPE states that "some of children's activity should be in periods lasting 10-15 minutes or more and include moderate to vigorous activity... alternating with brief periods of rest and recovery." Because children have difficulty tracking time on tasks, and because children's activity is intermittent in nature, we have opted to ask students to record what they did for activity, not how long.

   - The American Academy of Pediatrics recommends children and teens spend no more than two hours per day on leisure-time screen media: watching TV and movies and playing video and computer games.

6. IF YOU DO GOAL SETTING:

   - Help students be realistic about their goals. Physical activity must fit in with other daily activities and family schedules and must be safe and supervised according to family rules. Students don't need to trade all their excess Sit activity time for Fit activities. Trading 1-2 hours per week is probably realistic.

FitCheck Questions

Q. What kind of physical activities should students choose for a goal?

A. Whatever they like. They can select an activity to get better at, or they can pick an activity they are totally unfamiliar with and develop skills in that area.

Q. Do students have to choose a vigorous activity or a sport?

A. No. They can choose any physical activity to trade with their inactive time. This includes unstructured outdoor play.

Q. What happens if a student's goal is unmet by the next FitCheck?

A. The student can explore what prevented goal attainment in the Evaluation section. If this process is pursued in a non-critical fashion, it can help students modify their expectations and learn to set realistic goals.

Q. Is losing weight by the end of the school year a reasonable goal?

A. No. FitChecks should not be used as weight-loss tools. Many young people who think they need to lose weight really don't need to. Weight loss can be unhealthy while children are growing. Encourage children who want to lose weight to talk with their parents, the school nurse, and their physician.

FitCheck Journal

Adapted from Planet Health

Name _____ Date _____

Grade _____ FitCheck # _____

Start with today under Column 1, "Day of the week." Tonight you should do the following:

1. If you did any physical activities today, list them in column 2, and write a ✔ in column 3. Leave columns 2 and 3 blank if you did not do any physical activities today.

   • Include sports classes or practices, P.E. class, dance, or other active classes.

   • You can also list unstructured activities like running around with friends, pick-up sports, or active chores like raking or shoveling.

2. List today's TV and other "screen" activities in column 4. Estimate how much time these activities took in total. In column 5, write a ✔ if your total was two hours or less. Leave column 5 blank if your total was more than two hours.

   • Include TV shows, videos, movies, computer and video games, or surfing the Internet for fun.

   • Don't include using the computer for homework.

3. Do steps 1-2 for seven nights. Then, add up the number of ✔'s you have earned.

1. Day of the week	2. FitScore activities: sports, P.E., dance, games, free play, chores, etc.	3. Fit ✔'s	4. SitScore activities: TV, computer games, Internet surfing, videos, movies	5. Sit ✔'s
Total points	**FitScore**		**SitScore**	

Goal Setting

Name _____ Date _____

FitCheck # _____

What do your FitScore and SitScore mean? If your totals were 5-7, keep it up! If they were 0-4, TRY TO INCREASE THEM.

1. Your FitScore: _____   I need to (circle one):   Keep it up   Increase

2. Your SitScore: _____   I need to (circle one):   Keep it up   Increase

Make Fit and Sit goals! If you have scores you want to maintain, way to go! If you want to increase your scores, think of 1-3 realistic strategies you can work out with your family. For example, identify a time when you usually play computer games, and spend some or all of that time playing with friends or family instead. Or, walk or bike to school instead of getting a ride.

I will try to increase my (circle one or both)   FIT   SIT   scores by:

Goal Evaluation

Date _____

Did you meet your goals?

○ All of them
○ Some of them
○ None of them

Why/Why not? Write how you reached your goals, or why you did not reach them:

_____

_____

FitScore Progress Chart

Name _____

Find out how your FitScores change during the school year. Draw a bar for each FitScore in the first chart. Work from left to right. How have your scores changed?

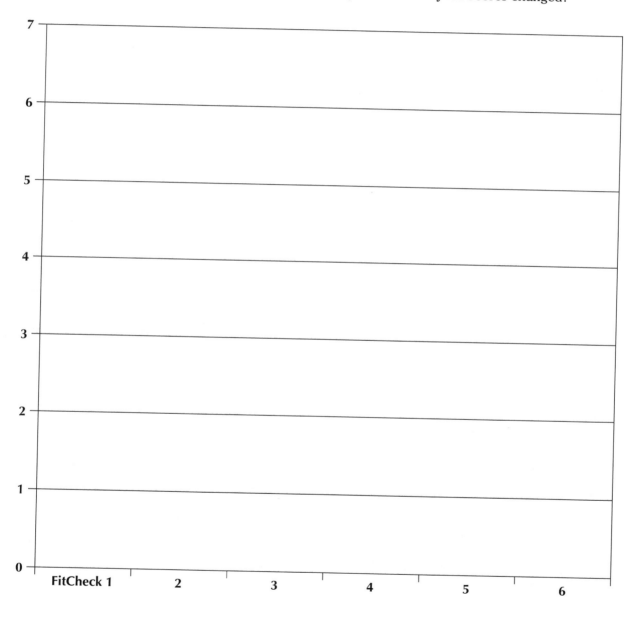

SitScore Progress Chart

Name _____

Find out how your SitScores change during the school year. Draw a bar for each SitScore in the chart. Work from left to right. How have your scores changed?

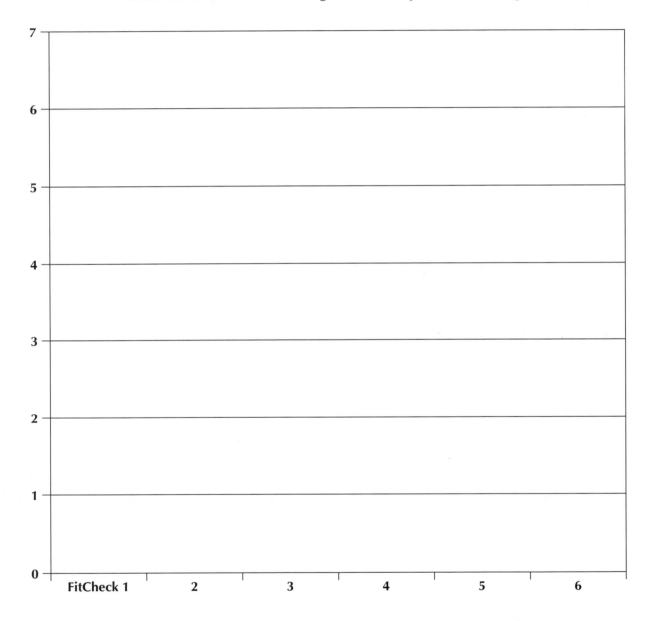

Students' Guide to the FitCheck

Fitness Tip

FitChecks will help you choose a healthy level of activity.

Fitness Lesson

[In this class/our next class] you will do a Planet Health FitCheck. The FitCheck is a way of keeping track of how much physical activity you're getting (time spent in moderate activities like walking and time spent in vigorous activities like running) as well as how much time you spend being inactive (time spent watching TV, playing video and computer games, and watching movies). Based on those measurements, you can create goals to increase or maintain your current level of activity.

You will take your FitCheck journal (see pp. 406-407) home to record your activities as a homework assignment during FitCheck weeks. After the FitCheck week comes to an end, you'll bring your FitCheck journal back to school where I'll keep it in/at[location at school] at all times. Only you will have access to your FitCheck journal. You will use the FitCheck journal two or three times during the school year.

To chart your progress, you will keep track of your activities for seven days, in and outside of school. You'll figure out how often you are physically active in P.E. class, sports teams or classes, dance classes, and other activities like active play with your friends and family, helping with leaves or snow, or big cleanup projects at home. You'll also figure out how much time you spend watching TV, playing computer games, and watching movies. The time you spend doing these non-physical activities represents time when you are not moving around.

At the end of the FitCheck week, you'll use your journal to figure out your FitScore and SitScore (see pp. 406-407). You'll graph these scores so that by the end of the year you'll see how your scores have changed.

A FitCheck consists of [*Teacher note: list the FitCheck components you have chosen to use*]:

1. Recording physical activities

2. Recording screen time (TV, computer games, videos, and movies)

3. Totaling your FitScore and SitScore at the end of the FitCheck week

4. Graphing your records

5. Setting goals

6. Evaluating progress toward goals (see p. 408)

FitCheck Physical Education Micro-Units

Part VI includes four micro-units that were developed specifically for the FitCheck—five-minute-long "brief lessons" that cover a wide range of physical activity topics. These micro-units were adapted from the middle-school curriculum, Planet Health*, and they are designed to build upon one another. The micro-units are best taught sequentially as a set. However, the micro-units can also be used intermittently—such as on days when no full-length Eat Well & *Keep Moving* physical education lesson is being taught—as long as the units are taught in the correct order.

The micro-units are formatted in a way to facilitate your delivery of their messages. The bulleted lists serve as key talking points that you can discuss with your students. The text boxes provide you with additional information that you may or may not want to cover during the five minutes. The How-To sections provide you with ideas to motivate your students on how they can accomplish the goals of the unit. Finally, the questions allow you to see how well your students picked up on the concepts of the lesson.

* Planet Health: Jill Carter, Jean Wiecha, Karen E. Peterson, and Steven L. Gortmaker, Human Kinetics, 2000.

Charting Your FitScore and SitScore

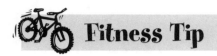

Fitness Tip

You can use the FitCheck Journal to find out how active you are.

Fitness Lesson

Using the FitCheck journal, you can chart your FitScore and SitScore:

- Your FitScore represents the time you were physically active during the past week. It is the number of points you earn for time spent participating in moderate and vigorous physical activities.

- Moderate physical activities include
  - stretching,
  - walking,
  - climbing on playground structures,
  - easy cycling,
  - easy swimming,
  - easy skating, and
  - light chores.

- Physical activities also include vigorous ones like
  - running,
  - tag games,
  - basketball,
  - soccer,
  - rope jumping,
  - roller blading,
  - fast cycling,
  - fast swimming, and
  - skating.

- Your SitScore represents the time you were not moving around during the past week. It is the total time you spent
  - watching TV,
  - playing computer games,
  - surfing the Internet for fun, and
  - watching videos and movies.

Defining Moderate and Vigorous Exercise Intensities

You should be able to talk easily while participating in an activity of light to moderate intensity.

Vigorous activities make you breathe hard and sweat.

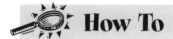

How To

Teachers, pass out a manila FitCheck journal and a pencil to each student. Go over the instructions, making sure students understand the assignment. Show them an example (you can use yourself as the example). Have them fill out the heading of the FitCheck journal. Then, read the following to your students:

1. At the end of the FitCheck week, each of you will figure out your scores.

   - For FitScores, you will get one point for every day when you listed at least one physical activity.

   - For SitScores, you will get one point for every day when your total time spent on "Sit" activities was two hours or less.

   - Aim for Fit- and SitScores of 5-7. If either score is between 0 and 4, you should set goals to improve your scores.

2. Now we will graph our scores.

Go over your own graphing instructions with your students at this time.

Questions for Students

1. What will your scores tell you about your lifestyle?

2. How might this journal change how you spend your free time?

What Could You Do Instead of Watching TV?

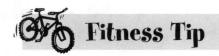

Fitness Tip

Watching less than 2 hours of TV each day can help you get fit!

Fitness Lesson

TV Cuts Down on Your Time to Be Active

- Many children your age spend a lot of their free time doing things that require sitting down.

- For some kids, this includes watching TV for about 5 hours a day.

- Think about how this cuts into your activity time.

Watching Too Much TV Can Make You Less Fit

- Being inactive day after day can quickly make you lose
  - flexibility,
  - muscle strength, and
  - cardiovascular endurance.

- When you sit still, you burn fewer calories than you would if you were moving around.

Watching Too Much TV Can Be Harmful to Your Health

When you sit in front of the TV, you lose a chance to be active and to improve your fitness level. Likewise, many people snack more than they need to while they are watching TV. Studies show that the kids who watch the least TV are the kids who are least likely to be overweight. The combination of eating too much and moving less can cause people to gain too much weight over time. People who are overweight are more likely to develop health problems, making it harder to lead a happy, active life.

420

Warning!!

Remember, you need plenty of healthy food for being active and growing, especially when you are growing fast. Never make a decision to cut back on the amount of food you eat without talking it over with your parents, your school nurse, or doctor.

How To

1. Doctors recommend that children and teens watch no more than 2 hours of TV each day.

2. This means you can watch up to 4 half-hour shows every day—but you can watch less, too.

3. Watch only shows you like.

4. Take note of the times when you watch TV but you aren't really interested—when you channel surf or watch reruns—and use that time to be physically active instead.

5. Try to limit your TV viewing to no more than 2 hours each day.

Questions for Students

1. What is the maximum amount of TV that doctors recommend children watch per day?

2. What could happen if you watch too much TV?

3. Why is being active better than watching TV, movies, or playing video games?

4. What are some activities that you can do instead of watching TV?

Making Time to Stay Fit

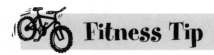

Fitness Tip

It's the regular in regular activity that's important. Make space for fitness!

Fitness Lesson

Making Space for Fitness

- Find the time to be active.
- Set aside a specific time to exercise.
- Small increases in physical activity add up over time, and can produce long-term health benefits.

Never Pass Up the Opportunity to Be Physically Active

- Stretch when you wake up in the morning.
- Take the stairs instead of the escalator or elevator at the mall.
- If it is safe for you, walk or bike instead of getting a ride or taking the bus.

Goal Setting

- It's important to set goals for increasing your physical activity.
- Today we will practice setting activity goals.
- We'll begin by trying to write a goal that will motivate each of you to be more active during today's class.

Exercise With Others

Exercising with others can make doing an activity more fun. Make a plan to exercise with a friend. You can also do active things you like with your parents, brothers, or sisters. Finally, you may want to join a team.

Finding Active Time at School

Think about times during the day when you can trade inactive time for physical activity. Try to be more active during PE, and walk briskly to your classes.

Finding Active Time Away From School

In addition, you can be more active while you are away from school. Invite friends over to play active games, practice dance, aerobics, or gymnastics. Clean your room (and your house). Vacuuming, cleaning out closets, and other tasks require bending, stretching, and lifting. Have fun with it! Listen to music!

Quick Ideas to Become More Fit

- Help a younger sister or brother get started in an activity or sport.
- Learn how to play with young children.
- Try to be as active as a two- or three-year-old—it just might tire you out.
- Watch TV only if it's your favorite show.
- Exercise while you watch your favorite shows on TV.
- Borrow an exercise video from the video store or library
- Take up an after-school activity or sport.
- Go for a walk or bike ride with a friend.
- Try to stay outside for an hour after school with your friends if your parents approve.

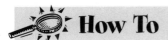 **How To**

Make one goal to be completed by all students in gym class today. For example, "I will warm up for 5 minutes before exercising, actively participate (break a sweat) in PE today, and spend 5 minutes cooling down at the end of class." You may want to discuss the goal with students and come up with one together.

1. Write the goal on the board (or in large print on sheets of paper hung on the wall), so students can see it throughout class.

2. At the end of class, leave time for students to evaluate whether they reached their goal.

3. Ask students the following:

   • Did you reach the class goal?

   • For those of you who reached the goal, how do you know you reached your goal?

   • For those of you who didn't reach your goal, what could you have done to reach your goal?

4. You may want to repeat this lesson in PE class until students are comfortable with goal setting and evaluation.

 ## Questions for Students

1. What are some ways you can make time to stay fit?

2. It's important to set realistic goals for yourself—ones that you have a reasonable chance of reaching. Which of the following goals is more realistic for a student who currently gets a ride to school from her mom? Goal 1: I will walk to and from school instead of getting a ride every day for the next month. Goal 2: I will walk to school three mornings a week for the next month.

Setting Goals for Personal Fitness

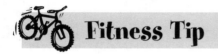

Fitness Tip

Set fitness goals that fit your life. Trade SIT time for FIT time.

If you have decided not to do goal-setting, you can skip this micro-unit.

Fitness Lesson

Setting Personal Fitness Goals

- Setting fitness goals is a good first step to getting fit.
- Today you will learn about goal setting.
- You will use the FitCheck sheet to set a personal fitness goal.
- While setting goals, keep in mind how much time you spent being inactive during the last FitCheck.

Trading Bored Time with Fun Time

How much of your time is spent

- channel surfing,
- watching shows you really don't like,
- watching reruns of shows you've already seen, and
- playing video games because you have nothing better to do?

That is the time you should trade for active time:

- Run around and play.
- Play a sport.
- Do an aerobics tape with a friend.
- Or take a walk with friends.

Eat Well & *Keep Moving* Fitness Goals

Elementary school-age children should get at least 30-60 minutes of activity from a variety of activities on all or most days of the week. Some of children's activity should be in periods lasting 10-15 minutes or more and include moderate to vigorous activity alternating with brief periods of rest and recovery (NASPE 1998). Children should spend no more than two hours per day watching TV and playing video or computer games.

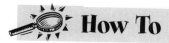 **How To**

Review the most recent FitCheck journals with your students. Make sure everyone has a pen or pencil. Read these instructions to students:

1. Review your most recent SitScore. Is it under 5? If yes, consider trading some Sit time for some Fit time.

2. Think about when you do your screen time: before school, after school, or before bed. When could you trade some for physical activity? Be specific! An example: after school on Mondays and Fridays I will skate, bike, or run around for a half hour instead of playing a computer game.

3. Choose activities you like! Fill in your goal with an activity you already do well, with a new activity you would like to try, or with an activity at which you would like to get better. Remember that making a plan with a friend could make it more fun and help you do it more often.

4. Make sure new activities are safe and supervised according to your family's rules. Make sure they fit in with your family's schedule.

Give students time to complete their goals, and then collect the journals and goal sheets.

Goal evaluation will be done during every FitCheck after the first. However, if this is your first time doing the FitCheck with your class, then please proceed to the Questions for Students.

Goal Evaluation

Evaluating the previous goal will be the first thing you do in a FitCheck, beginning with the second FitCheck.

1. Put today's date in the Evaluation section's date box.

2. Read your goal from the previous FitCheck you did.

3. Check "yes" or "no" to answer the question, "Did you meet your goal?"

4. In one or two sentences, explain how you reached your goal, or why you did not reach your goal.

 ## Questions for Students

1. Why should you trade some of your inactive time for active time?

2. Are there times that you watch TV shows that you don't like, or that you channel surf or watch reruns (shows you have already seen) simply because you are bored? Could you do some physical activity instead of being bored?

Additional Physical Education Micro-Units

Part VII includes five additional micro-units—five-minute-long "brief lessons" that cover a wide range of physical activity topics. These micro-units were adapted from the middle-school curriculum, Planet Health*, and they are designed to build upon one another. The micro-units are best taught sequentially as a set. However, the micro-units can also be used intermittently—such as on days when no full-length Eat Well & *Keep Moving* physical education lesson is being taught—as long as the units are taught in the correct order.

The micro-units are formatted in a way to facilitate your delivery of their messages. The bulleted lists serve as key talking points that you can discuss with your students. The text boxes provide you with additional information that you may or may not want to cover during the five minutes. The How-To sections provide you with ideas to motivate your students on how they can accomplish the goals of the unit. Finally, the questions allow you to see how well your students picked up on the concepts of the lesson.

* Planet Health: Jill Carter, Jean Wiecha, Karen E. Peterson, and Steven L. Gortmaker, Human Kinetics, 2000.

Thinking About Activity, Exercise, and Fitness

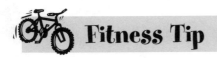

Any physical activity is better than none.

Fitness Lesson

A Brief Introduction to Physical Fitness

- Being fit means you have the energy you need to
  - work,
  - exercise,
  - play, and
  - get from place to place without easily tiring.
- To get fit, you need to be physically active.

Be Active and Eat Right

- Exercise is physical activity that is planned and structured, like running a mile or playing soccer for an hour. Many people think that only exercise improves fitness.
- In fact, many kinds of movement can improve your health and fitness level:
  - Dancing
  - Jumping rope
  - Walking the dog
  - Throwing a ball
  - Climbing stairs
  - Swimming
- But, the more active you are, the more fit you will become.
- In addition to physical activity, healthy eating will also help you stay fit.
- We'll discuss more about this aspect of fitness later.

Positive Effects of Physical Fitness

- Being physically fit
  - makes you healthier,
  - helps you build a positive self-image, and
  - helps you feel better about yourself.
- Fitness is fun, and it feels great!

Long-Term Health Benefits of Physical Activity

Learning to be active now will help you become an active adult. If you become fit now and stay active as you get older, you'll lower your risk of having certain health problems as an adult, such as obesity, heart disease, broken bones, bone loss, diabetes, and certain types of cancers. Moderate amounts of physical activity will help you prevent these health problems.

Physical Activity Recommendations for Children

Elementary school-age children should accumulate at least 30-60 minutes of activity from a variety of activities on all or most days of the week. Some of children's activity should be in periods lasting 10-15 minutes or more and include moderate to vigorous activity . . . alternating with brief periods of rest and recovery (NASPE 1998).

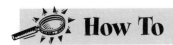 **How To**

1. Start thinking about the physical activities that you do and the things you do that are not active, like

   - watching TV,

   - playing video and computer games, and

   - watching movies.

2. Next, think about ways to increase your activity level. You can do this by replacing inactive time with active time. For instance, you can

   - ride bikes instead of watching a show on TV that you don't really like, and

   - play basketball instead of playing a video game.

3. Remember, being active will help you stay healthy now, and as you grow up.

Questions for Students

1. What are some of the things that you do to be physically active?
2. What can you do to increase your physical activity?
3. What are the benefits of being fit?
4. What kinds of things get in the way of your being more physically active?

Be Active Now for a Healthy Heart Later

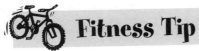

Being active in your free time now can lower your risk of cardiovascular disease later in life.

Fitness Lesson

The Number One Killer

- Cardiovascular disease is a disease of the heart and blood vessels.
- It is the single largest cause of death in the United States for both men and women.

Preventing the Number One Killer

- You can lower your risk of developing cardiovascular disease by starting a lifelong commitment to regular exercise now.
- Maintaining a healthy weight, eating a balanced diet that is low in saturated fat and moderate in total fat, and living smoke-free will also help you prevent cardiovascular disease.

Cardiovascular Disease in the United States

Cardiovascular disease is actually a group of diseases that affect the heart and blood vessels. It includes coronary artery disease (a narrowing of the arteries in the heart that can cause a heart attack, chest pain, or both), stroke, rheumatic heart disease, and many others. According to 1996 estimates, 58,800,000 Americans have one or more forms of cardiovascular disease. A total of 959,227 Americans died from cardiovascular disease in 1996 (41.1% of all deaths).

Habits That Put Adults at Risk for Cardiovascular Disease Begin in the Teens

Overeating, feeling stressed, eating high-fat (saturated and *trans*) diets, being inactive (not moving around), and smoking are all habits that could lead to being overweight, having high blood cholesterol, and developing other factors that cause cardiovascular disease.

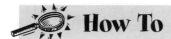 **How To**

1. To prevent cardiovascular disease, develop good physical activity and eating habits at an early age and maintain them throughout your life.

2. Choose activities that make your heart and lungs stronger, like

   - fast walking,
   - running,
   - bicycling,
   - swimming,
   - in-line skating, and
   - hiking.

3. Eat at least five fruits and vegetables a day and a diet low in saturated and *trans* fats and moderate in total fat.

4. Finally, don't smoke!

 Questions for Students

1. Name some physical activities that you like to do that will strengthen your heart.

2. Which of these activities do you think you will continue as an adult?

Be Active Now for Healthy Bones Later

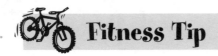

Fitness Tip

Building strong bones now can help prevent fractures and bone loss later in life.

 ## Fitness Lesson

Building Strong Bones

- Almost 50% of your bone mass is formed during your childhood and teen years.

- Exercising and eating a balanced diet rich in calcium and vitamin D will help you build strong bones.

- Building strong bones now is a critical part of preventing osteoporosis from developing when you are older.

- Living a healthy lifestyle with no smoking and limited alcohol consumption during adulthood will keep your bones strong.

- People with osteoporosis have weak bones that are more likely to break. For example, hip fractures are common among the elderly and are a serious injury because older peoples' bones do not heal easily.

Building Strong Bones With Exercise

- Weight-bearing exercises build strong bones.

- In weight-bearing exercises, your bones and muscles work against gravity; your feet, legs, or arms support your weight as you move. Some examples of this kind of activity are
  - walking,
  - stair climbing,
  - hiking,
  - racket sports,
  - dancing,
  - soccer,
  - push-ups,
  - curl-ups, and
  - basketball, but
  - *not* swimming or biking.

- Weight training also builds strong bones.

- Hitting a ball or landing on your feet after jumping stimulates more calcium to be deposited in your bone. More calcium makes your bones stronger.

- Most sports and daily physical activities require weight-bearing activities. If you participate regularly in a variety of physical activities, you will build strong bones.

Osteoporosis

Osteoporosis literally means "porous bone." While the shape of the bones looks okay, they have fewer minerals in them. The minerals calcium and phosphorus are the major building blocks of bone. Bones that are low in these minerals are brittle and break more easily than healthy bones. It is estimated that 15 to 20 million Americans suffer from osteoporosis. Osteoporosis is more common among women than men (roughly 80% of osteoporosis cases are in women).

Preventing Osteoporosis Also Requires Consuming Enough Calcium

In order to prevent osteoporosis, you need to make sure that you are consuming enough calcium. Persons 9-18 years old require 1,300 milligrams of calcium per day, the amount found in four 8-ounce glasses of milk. Milk and other dairy products (yogurt, cheese) offer the largest amount of calcium per serving. Other excellent sources of calcium include

- tofu,
- sardines with bones,
- calcium-fortified foods including orange juice, cereal, and cereal bars.

Spinach, broccoli, and other green leafy vegetables are good sources of calcium, but provide a lot fewer grams per serving than most milk products. If you are unable to consume milk or milk products, you should eat other calcium-rich foods.

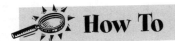

How To

1. To build strong bones and prevent osteoporosis, develop good exercise and eating habits now.

2. Choose physical activities that put some stress on your bones.

3. Eat foods rich in calcium. Have four servings of low-fat dairy products like milk, cheese, and yogurt every day.

Questions for Students

1. How does exercise help your bones?

2. How can you help prevent osteoporosis and bone fractures?

Let's Get Started on Being Fit

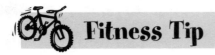

Fitness Tip

For total physical fitness, work on cardiovascular endurance, muscle strength, and flexibility.

Fitness Lesson

Understanding Physical Fitness

- Being physically fit means you have the energy and strength to handle the everyday demands of your life:
  - A walk to school
  - A game of soccer during gym
  - Actively listening and participating in class
  - Completing daily chores
  - Participating in after-school activities
  - Doing a good job on your homework
  - Sprinting to escape the jaws of the neighborhood dog
- You can complete all of your daily activities without feeling overly fatigued.

Overall Physical Fitness

- Many factors contribute to your overall physical fitness.
- The factors that are most important to your health are
  1. cardiovascular endurance (or cardiovascular fitness),
  2. muscle strength, and
  3. flexibility.

The Three Areas of Physical Fitness

- Physical fitness consists of cardiovascular endurance, muscle strength, and flexibility. Each one of these components helps your body to be physically fit in different ways.
- Cardiovascular endurance helps you do physical work or play for a long time without getting tired. This requires your heart, blood vessels, lungs, and muscles to efficiently carry and use oxygen.
- Muscle strength helps you lift and move yourself and heavy stuff.
- Flexibility helps you reach, bend, twist, and move without injury.

Bone Integrity and Body Composition Are Two Other Components of Health-Related Fitness

Regular physical activity will help you build strong bones and maintain a healthy body composition. A fit person has strong bones and muscles and a healthy amount of body fat.

Skill-Related Components of Physical Fitness

Success in sports and other physical activities may require you to develop some other abilities, such as

- agility,
- balance,
- power,
- speed,
- coordination, and
- reaction time.

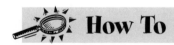 **How To**

1. To improve your cardiovascular endurance, do physical activities that increase your heart and breathing rate:

    - Walk briskly
    - Hike
    - Swim
    - Play dodge ball
    - Jump rope
    - Play soccer
    - Dance

- Ride your bike
- Do in-line skating

2. To improve your strength and muscular endurance, do work, play, or exercise that makes you repeatedly lift or move a load (an object, your body, a weight) that is heavier than you are used to.

   - Do push-ups, pull-ups, and sit-ups.
   - Pedal your bike up an incline.
   - Shovel snow.

3. Performing these activities in sets of repetitions will improve your muscle strength and endurance.

4. To improve your flexibility, stretch regularly. Activities like gymnastics, dance, and figure skating require good flexibility.

5. To best improve your overall physical fitness, participate in a variety of physical activities.

6. Be sure to do activities that work and stretch the upper and lower body parts.

Questions for Students

1. Can you name some activities that will improve each component of physical fitness?

2. Which area of fitness do you think you need to improve the most?

More About the Three Areas of Physical Fitness

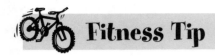

Fitness Tip

To get fit, choose a mixture of activities that you can do regularly to build your cardiovascular endurance, muscle strength, and flexibility.

Fitness Lesson

Physical Fitness

- We learned that in order to be physically fit and to meet the daily demands of work and play, a person must possess an adequate level of

  - cardiovascular endurance,

  - muscular strength, and

  - flexibility.

- To be fit, you need to work in all three areas of fitness because each area has a different effect on your body.

Some Activities Address One Area of Fitness, While Others Address More Than One

- To be fit, you need to participate in a variety of physical activities.

- It is important that you be able to identify which activities belong to different fitness areas.

- Then you need to identify activities in each area that you enjoy and do them.

No One Type of Physical Activity Improves All Components of Fitness

Aerobic activities generally increase cardiovascular and muscle endurance, but not strength and flexibility. Similarly, many activities that build muscular strength and flexibility don't do much for endurance. These activities only improve the body part being worked. Therefore, strength and flexibility exercises must be performed by each muscle group and at each joint.

450

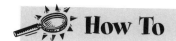 **How To**

1. Let's think about some daily activities and exercises you do, and figure out what areas of physical fitness they address. For example: what area of physical fitness do you work on when you

   - carry heavy boxes or grocery bags? (improves upper-body strength),

   - bike to your friend's house? (increases your cardiovascular endurance), and

   - shovel snow? (improves muscle strength and endurance and cardiovascular endurance).

Ask students to name a few activities. Involve the class in identifying the components of physical fitness being addressed.

 Questions for Students

1. Name three components of physical fitness.

2. Which component do you need to work on the most?

3. During class today we will play (or do) [activity]. What components of fitness will we be working on during this activity?

Appendix

The Stretches

Stretching positions are the same for all people. However, the extent of the stretch depends on the flexibility of the individual. Safety is important, so stretches should not be taken beyond comfortable levels. Ten to fifteen seconds is the recommended time to hold each stretch.

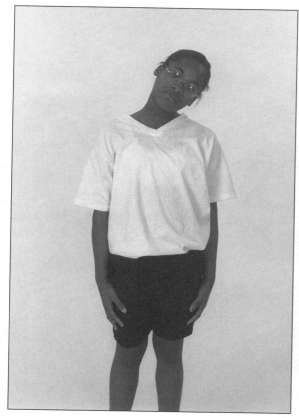

Neck stretch

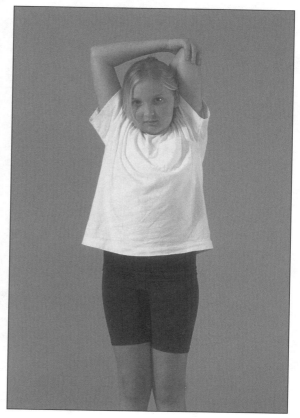

Arm and shoulder stretch

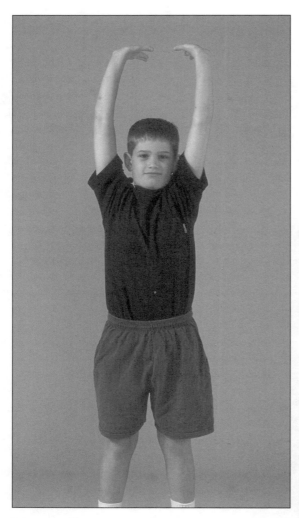

Palms to ceiling

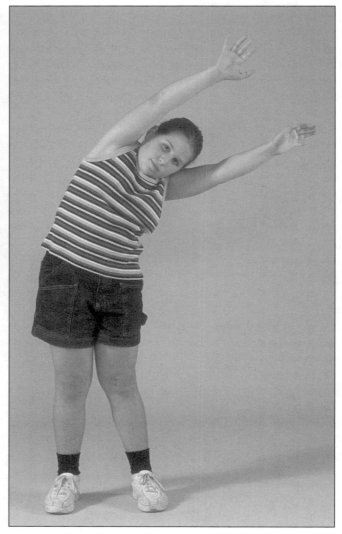

The wave

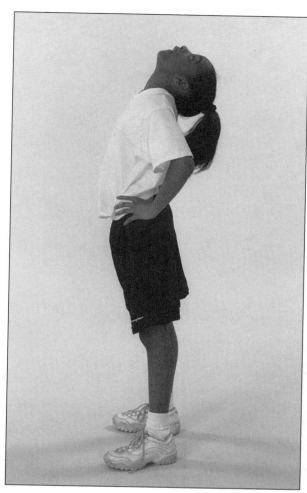

Reach back

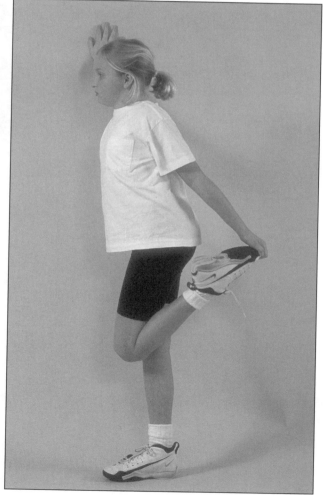

Quad burner

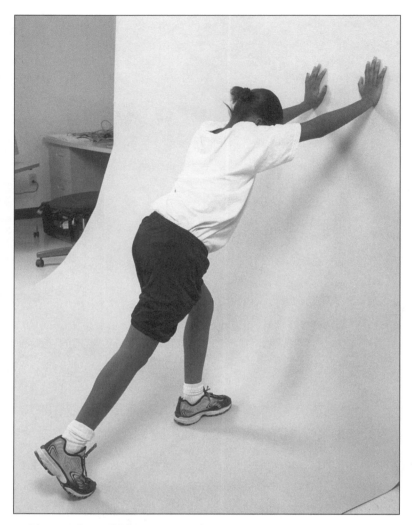

Holding up the wall hamstring stretch

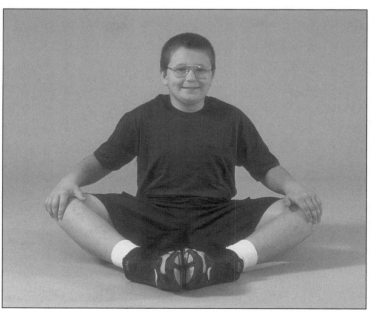

Butterfly

Strength Fitness Diagrams

Upper-Body Strength

Regular Push-Ups

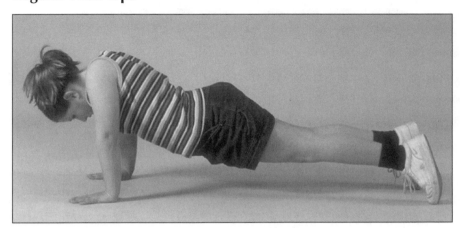

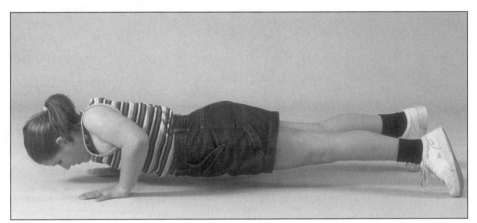

Modified Push-Ups

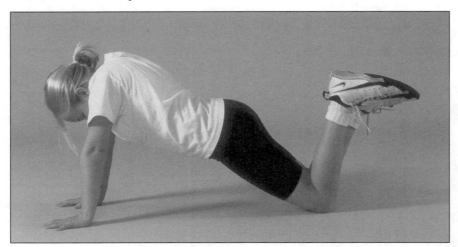

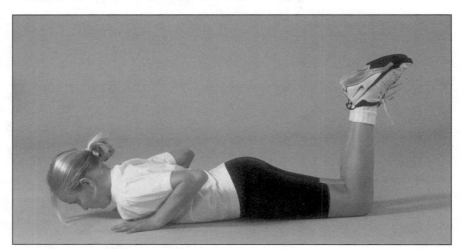

Stomach Strength

Abdominal Crunches

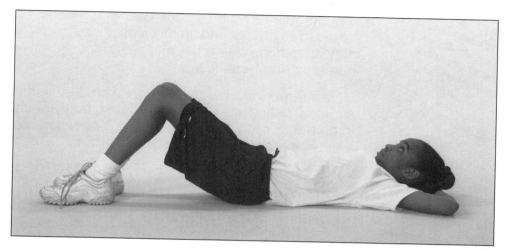

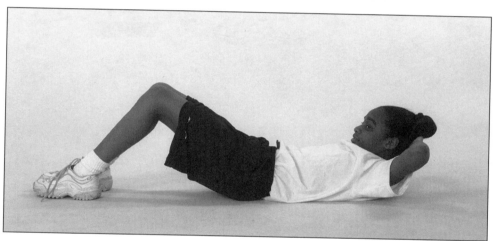

Stir-Fry Without the Fat!

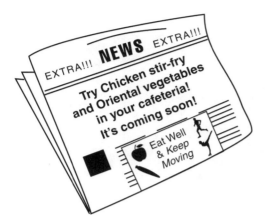

Stir-fry means to cook over high heat, briskly stirring the ingredients so they cook evenly. Because the vegetables are cut into small pieces, they cook quickly, stay crispy and delicious, and retain most of their nutrients and fresh flavor.

Unlike deep-fried foods (fried chicken, for example) stir-fried dishes are low in fat because they are cooked in non-stick pans with only a tiny bit of vegetable oil and/or another liquid, like chicken broth.

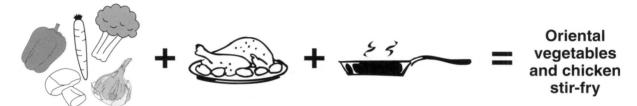

Oriental vegetables and chicken stir-fry

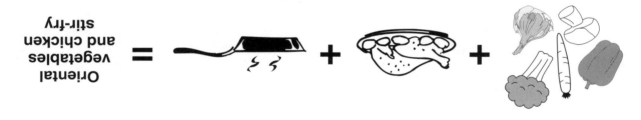

Stir-Fry Without the Fat!

Stir-fry means to cook over high heat, briskly stirring the ingredients so they cook evenly. Because the vegetables are cut into small pieces, they cook quickly, stay crispy and delicious, and retain most of their nutrients and fresh flavor.

Unlike deep-fried foods (fried chicken, for example) stir-fried dishes are low in fat because they are cooked in non-stick pans with only a tiny bit of vegetable oil and/or another liquid, like chicken broth.

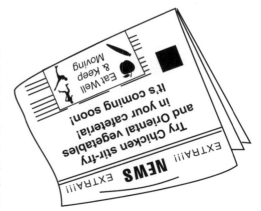

What's the New Food?
Chunky Vegetable Stew

What's in the Chunky Vegetable Stew?

Tomatoes

Tomatoes have lots of vitamin C to help you heal cuts and scrapes. Vitamin C can also help you fight off colds and flus.

Carrots

Carrots have a lot of vitamin A, which helps keep your bones strong and eyesight good.

Potatoes

Potatoes are packed with energy to help you run, dance, and think. They also have potassium, which is very important for working muscles.

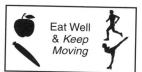

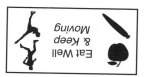

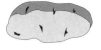

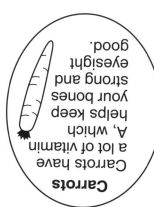

Potatoes are packed with energy to help you run, dance, and think. They also have potassium, which is very important for working muscles.

Carrots have a lot of vitamin A, which helps keep your bones strong and eyesight good.

Tomatoes have lots of vitamin C to help you heal cuts and scrapes. Vitamin C can also help you fight off colds and flus.

Potatoes **Carrots** **Tomatoes**

What's in the Chunky Vegetable Stew?

Chunky Vegetable Stew
What's the New Food?

To Nourish Your Body As Well As Your Soul…
5-A-Day Should Be Your Goal!

Bell pepper

Pear

Fruits and vegetables are not only colorful and naturally beautiful, they are also packed with vitamins, minerals, and fiber. Research has even shown that they can reduce the risk of certain forms of cancer.

The Food Guide Pyramid recommends that we eat 2-3 servings of fruit every day and 3-4 servings of veggies every day.

So, if you don't already eat at least 5 servings of fruits and vegetables each day, give it a try. It will do wonders for your health!

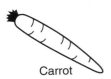

Carrot

Tomato

Apple

Grapes

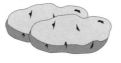

Potatoes

Eggplant

Eggplant

Potatoes

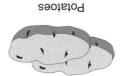

Grapes

Apple

So, if you don't already eat at least 5 servings of fruits and vegetables each day, give it a try. It will do wonders for your health!

Tomato

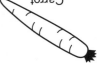

Carrot

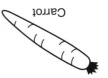

The Food Guide Pyramid recommends that we eat 2-3 servings of fruit every day and 3-4 servings of veggies every day.

Fruits and vegetables are not only colorful and naturally beautiful, they are also packed with vitamins, minerals, and fiber. Research has even shown that they can reduce the risk of certain forms of cancer.

Pear

Bell pepper

5-A-Day Should Be Your Goal!
To Nourish Your Body As Well As Your Soul…

Low-Fat Milk…"The Perfect Food"

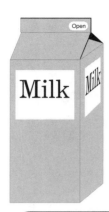

Low-fat milk, *an important part of the dairy group in the Food Guide Pyramid,* could be called "the perfect food."

Do you know why?

Because it contains all the nutrients needed to help you grow and keep you healthy. Low-fat milk and foods made from low-fat milk (like low-fat cheese, yogurt, and ice cream) provide your body with calcium, protein, carbohydrates, vitamins, and, of course, very little fat!

😊 Smile!

Did you know that the calcium in milk is great for helping to keep your teeth healthy and strong?

Calcium is important for all of the growing bones in your body. So drink milk, smile…and show off those pearly whites!

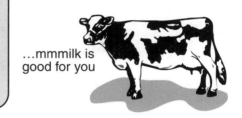

…mmmilk is good for you

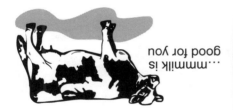

…mmmilk is good for you

😊 Smile!

Did you know that the calcium in milk is great for helping to keep your teeth healthy and strong?

Calcium is important for all of the growing bones in your body. So drink milk, smile…and show off those pearly whites!

Because it contains all the nutrients needed to help you grow and keep you healthy. Low-fat milk and foods made from low-fat milk (like low-fat cheese, yogurt, and ice cream) provide your body with calcium, protein, carbohydrates, vitamins, and, of course, very little fat!

Do you know why?

Low-fat milk, *an important part of the dairy group in the Food Guide Pyramid,* could be called "the perfect food."

Low-Fat Milk…"The Perfect Food"

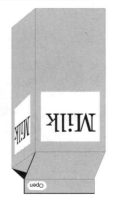

Oranges for Each Day's Journey

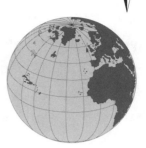

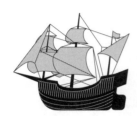 Oranges originally grew in Asia and the East Indies (do you know where these are on the map?) and were brought to Europe by explorers and then to the New World (North America).

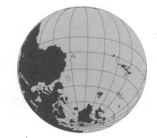 The vitamin C in oranges and other citrus fruit (like lemons, limes, and grapefruit) helped to keep these early explorers, like Columbus, Magellan, and Marco Polo, healthy on their very long journeys across the seas. Just like the explorers, you can keep healthy and strong on your daily journeys (to school, home, and the store) by eating oranges and other citrus. It's as easy as pouring a glass of 100% juice or eating the orange wedges served in the cafeteria. You'll be energized to play, and the vitamin C will help you grow strong, heal cuts and bruises, and fight off infections.

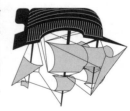

The vitamin C in oranges and other citrus fruit (like lemons, limes, and grapefruit) helped to keep these early explorers, like Columbus, Magellan, and Marco Polo, healthy on their very long journeys across the seas. Just like the explorers, you can keep healthy and strong on your daily journeys (to school, home, and the store) by eating oranges and other citrus. It's as easy as pouring a glass of 100% juice or eating the orange wedges served in the cafeteria. You'll be energized to play, and the vitamin C will help you grow strong, heal cuts and bruises, and fight off infections.

Oranges originally grew in Asia and the East Indies (do you know where these are on the map?) and were brought to Europe by explorers and then to the New World (North America).

Oranges for Each Day's Journey

Can you tell the difference between 100% fruit juice and regular fruit punch?

Easy! Only the pure juice will say "100% juice" right on the label–this goes for orange juice, grapefruit juice, or any kind of juice, really.

So why should you care whether it's 100% juice? Because, in addition to tasting great, 100% juice is packed with vitamins and minerals. Take the 100% orange juice you can get for breakfast in the cafeteria: it contains vitamin C and potassium that helps your body heal cuts and keeps your muscles working great.

Other fruit drinks and colored punches that don't say "100%" on the label may look like pure juice, but they usually contain very little juice (often none at all) and a lot of sugar. And 100% juice is the only drink that counts toward your 5-a-day for fruits and vegetables. So for your body and for your health:

GET YOUR BOOST FROM 100% JUICE

Open

100% Juice

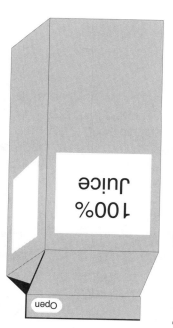

GET YOUR BOOST FROM 100% JUICE

vegetables. So for your body and for your health: is the only drink that counts toward your 5-a-day for fruits and juice little juice (often none at all) and a lot of sugar. And 100% the label may look like pure juice, but they usually contain very Other fruit drinks and colored punches that don't say "100%" on

your body heal cuts and keeps your muscles working great. in the cafeteria: it contains vitamin C and potassium that helps minerals. Take the 100% orange juice you can get for breakfast addition to tasting great, 100% juice is packed with vitamins and So why should you care whether it's 100% juice? Because, in

grapefruit juice, or any kind of juice, really. right on the label–this goes for orange juice, Easy! Only the pure juice will say "100% juice"

100% Juice

Open

Can you tell the difference between 100% fruit juice and regular fruit punch?

Have You Ever Heard of Pineapple Oranges?
How About Valencia, Temple, Navel, or Blood Oranges?

The oranges you usually see in the cafeteria are called pineapple oranges. These are popular because they have few seeds and have the familiar bright orange skin.

All types of oranges are sweet and juicy, but each has a different name and looks a little bit different from one another. Some are light orange on the inside, some are bright orange on the inside, and some are even bright red (these are called blood oranges).

Some have thin skin and some have thick skin. They also come in different sizes, ranging from the smaller temple to the larger navel.

Because oranges are so delicious, they make a great snack–even a sweet dessert! You can eat them peeled or cut into wedges, like in the cafeteria, or you can "drink" them as 100% juice. Any of these ways lets you enjoy oranges and gives you a boost of vitamin C that helps you grow, play, and learn.

Have You Ever Heard of Pineapple Oranges?
How About Valencia, Temple, Navel, or Blood Oranges?

The oranges you usually see in the cafeteria are called pineapple oranges. These are popular because they have few seeds and have the familiar bright orange skin.

All types of oranges are sweet and juicy, but each has a different name and looks a little bit different from one another. Some are light orange on the inside, some are bright orange on the inside, and some are even bright red (these are called blood oranges).

Some have thin skin and some have thick skin. They also come in different sizes, ranging from the smaller temple to the larger navel.

Because oranges are so delicious, they make a great snack–even a sweet dessert! You can eat them peeled or cut into wedges, like in the cafeteria, or you can "drink" them as 100% juice. Any of these ways lets you enjoy oranges and gives you a boost of vitamin C that helps you grow, play, and learn.

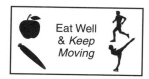

Have a Little Slice of Spring

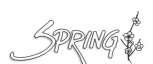

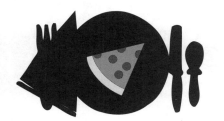

Pri•ma•ve•ra *adjective*

1: Made with different kinds of sliced or diced vegetables
2: From Latin, meaning "early spring" (**primus** = first + **ver** = spring)

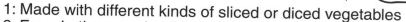

The word "primavera" can be traced back to the Latin roots *primus*, meaning "first," and *ver*, meaning "spring." Some springtime vegetables you may find in a primavera dish (pasta primavera or pizza primavera, for example) are peas, green beans, tomatoes, asparagus, and mushrooms. But don't be surprised if you find other kinds of vegetables in your primavera, like broccoli, onions, or carrots. Great chefs like to be creative!

This winter, when you're dreaming of warmer days, have some Pizza Primavera for lunch. It's like having a little slice of spring! And it's coming to your cafeteria soon!

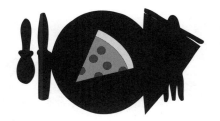

This winter, when you're dreaming of warmer days, have some Pizza Primavera for lunch. It's like having a little slice of spring! And it's coming to your cafeteria soon!

The word "primavera" can be traced back to the Latin roots *primus*, meaning "first," and *ver*, meaning "spring." Some springtime vegetables you may find in a primavera dish (pasta primavera or pizza primavera, for example) are peas, green beans, tomatoes, asparagus, and mushrooms. But don't be surprised if you find other kinds of vegetables in your primavera, like broccoli, onions, or carrots. Great chefs like to be creative!

Pri•ma•ve•ra *adjective*

1: Made with different kinds of sliced or diced vegetables
2: From Latin, meaning "early spring" (**primus** = first + **ver** = spring)

Have a Little Slice of Spring

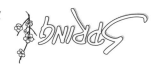

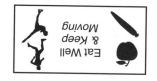

What a Treat to Eat a Sweet Peach!

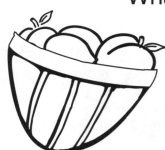

Peaches are rich in vitamins and minerals, especially vitamin A and potassium. They also contain iron, niacin, and vitamin C.

The peach originated in China around 2000 B.C. and was regarded as a symbol of life. Peaches are still used to help celebrate birthdays in China. A special peach dessert is often served at Chinese birthday parties.

Fresh peaches are best tasting and most available in the summer, but you can eat canned or frozen peaches all year around! They are delicious for breakfast, as a snack, or for dessert. Eat them by themselves, sliced with other fruit or on cereal, or bake them into a pie or crispy dessert.

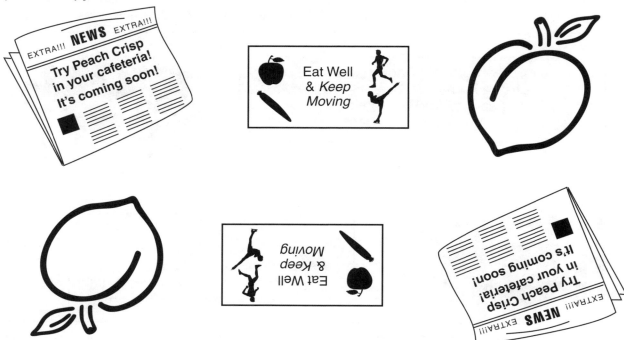

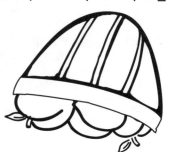

Potatoes

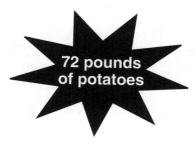

72 pounds of potatoes

That's the amount of potatoes the average person in the United States eats every year, and each pound is packed with energy and vitamin C.

They're good for you, and they taste great!

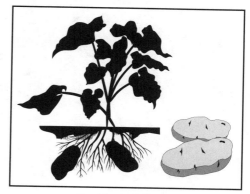

Picture of potatoes growing in the ground.

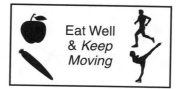

Eat Well & *Keep Moving*

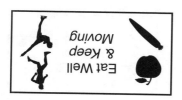

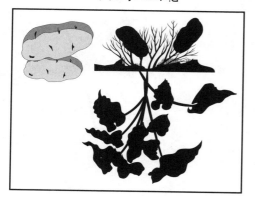

Picture of potatoes growing in the ground.

Eat Well & *Keep Moving*

That's the amount of potatoes the average person in the United States eats every year, and each pound is packed with energy and vitamin C.

They're good for you, and they taste great!

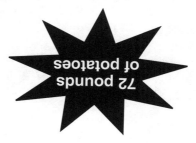

72 pounds of potatoes

Potatoes

A Message From Bobby Broccoli

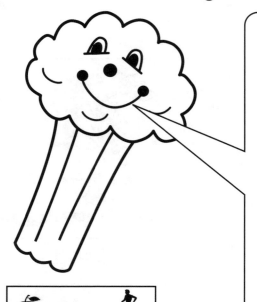

Hi kids! My name is Bobby Broccoli and I would like to fill you in on (and up with) some tasty tidbits of news…

- According to a poll by the EPCOT Center in Florida, broccoli and its family member, cauliflower, ranked #1 for "favorite veggies."

- Broccoli has been called the #1 anti-cancer vegetable. It is loaded with vitamin C and fiber, is very low in fat, and is rich in carotene—a nutrient that is believed to help prevent cancer.

- Broccoli is a terrific vegetable source of calcium. It's good for your teeth and bones!

I know we're going to like each other!

P.S. Try steamed broccoli in your cafeteria!

Eat Well & *Keep Moving*

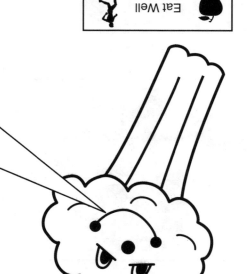

A Message From Bobby Broccoli

Hi kids! My name is Bobby Broccoli and I would like to fill you in on (and up with) some tasty tidbits of news…

- According to a poll by the EPCOT Center in Florida, broccoli and its family member, cauliflower, ranked #1 for "favorite veggies."

- Broccoli has been called the #1 anti-cancer vegetable. It is loaded with vitamin C and fiber, is very low in fat, and is rich in carotene—a nutrient that is believed to help prevent cancer.

- Broccoli is a terrific vegetable source of calcium. It's good for your teeth and bones!

I know we're going to like each other!

P.S. Try steamed broccoli in your cafeteria!

Eat Well & *Keep Moving*

What's the New Food?
Sweet Potatoes and Orange Juice

Sweet potatoes contain a lot of vitamin A, which is needed for strong bones and good eyesight. They also give you energy for playing and learning.

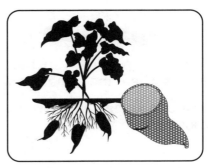

Picture of sweet potatoes growing in the ground and in cross-section.

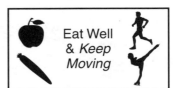

Eat Well & *Keep Moving*

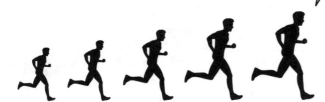

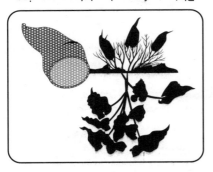

Eat Well & *Keep Moving*

Picture of sweet potatoes growing in the ground and in cross-section.

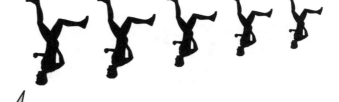

Sweet potatoes contain a lot of vitamin A, which is needed for strong bones and good eyesight. They also give you energy for playing and learning.

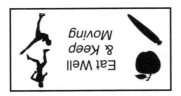

What's the New Food?
Sweet Potatoes and Orange Juice

That's One Sweet Potato!

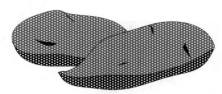

Sweet potatoes contain a lot of vitamin A, which is needed for strong bones, fighting infections, and good eyesight. In general, fruits and vegetables that are orange (like sweet potatoes and carrots) are a great source of vitamin A.

The sweet potato is very hardy and grows underground. It grows especially well in southern states where the climate is warm.

Sweet potatoes are a sweet, delicious, and nutritious addition to many meals. Try some today!

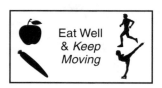

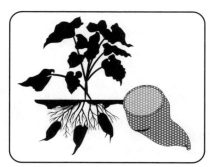

Picture of sweet potatoes growing in the ground and in cross-section.

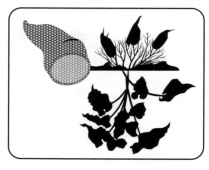

Picture of sweet potatoes growing in the ground and in cross-section.

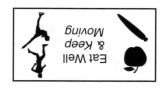

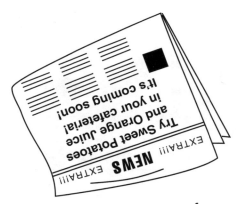

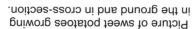

Sweet potatoes are a sweet, delicious, and nutritious addition to many meals. Try some today!

states where the climate is warm.

The sweet potato is very hardy and grows underground. It grows especially well in southern

potatoes and carrots) are a great source of vitamin A.

general, fruits and vegetables that are orange (like sweet for strong bones, fighting infections, and good eyesight. In Sweet potatoes contain a lot of vitamin A, which is needed

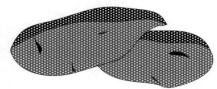

That's One Sweet Potato!

The Power of Pasta!

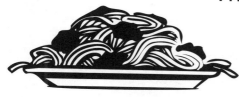

Because runners know that pasta is a terrific energy source, it is the traditional meal before big races. In fact, all runners in the Boston Marathon are treated to a spaghetti dinner the night before the race.

The good word about pasta's benefits has begun to spread among athletes in all sports. Even football coaches, who in the past have fed their teams big steak dinners before games, are changing the pre-game meal to…guess what? Pasta!

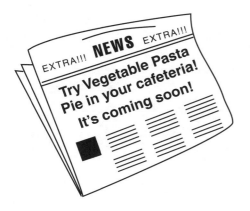

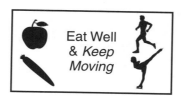

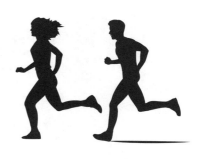

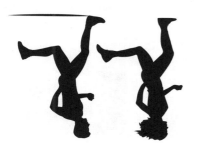

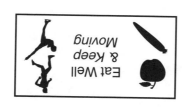

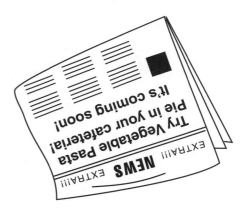

The good word about pasta's benefits has begun to spread among athletes in all sports. Even football coaches, who in the past have fed their teams big steak dinners before games, are changing the pre-game meal to…guess what? Pasta!

Because runners know that pasta is a terrific energy source, it is the traditional meal before big races. In fact, all runners in the Boston Marathon are treated to a spaghetti dinner the night before the race.

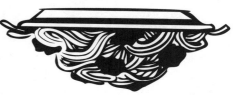

The Power of Pasta!

What's the New Food?
Vegetable Spaghetti Salad

Do you know where spaghetti came from originally?

You might think Italy, but, actually, spaghetti may have first come from China.

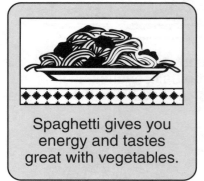

Spaghetti gives you energy and tastes great with vegetables.

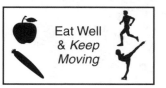

Eat Well & *Keep Moving*

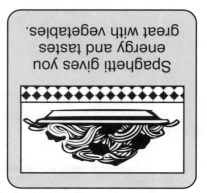

Spaghetti gives you energy and tastes great with vegetables.

Eat Well & *Keep Moving*

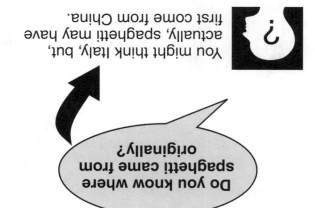

You might think Italy, but, actually, spaghetti may have first come from China.

Do you know where spaghetti came from originally?

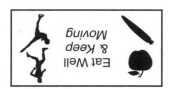

What's the New Food?
Vegetable Spaghetti Salad

Pasta Trivia!

Thomas Jefferson played a role in introducing pasta to this country. While serving as an ambassador to France in the late 1700s, Jefferson traveled to Naples, Italy, and was so impressed with the pasta he sampled that he had crates of it sent back to the U.S. along with a pasta-making machine.

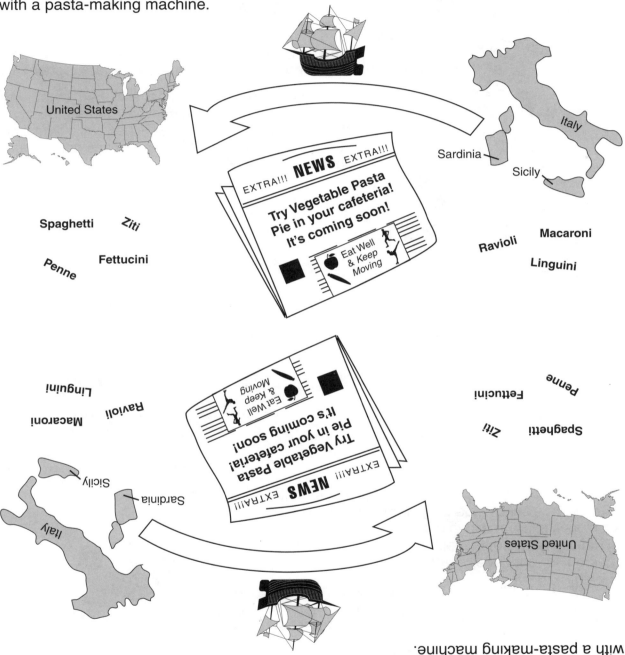

Whole Wheat Bread vs. White Bread

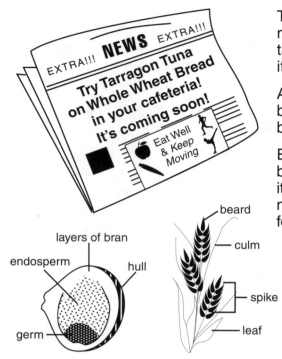

Try the wonderful world of whole wheat bread! It may look a little different, but whole wheat bread tastes good and is good for you. The more you eat it, the more you'll like it!

And it's more nutritious than white bread. White bread is made from wheat flour, which has had the bran and wheat germ removed from the grain.

Even when the white flour is "enriched" by adding back nutrients, only 4 nutrients are added. Compare it to whole wheat flour–the enriched white flour lacks much of the fiber and 18 other vitamins and minerals found in whole wheat flour.

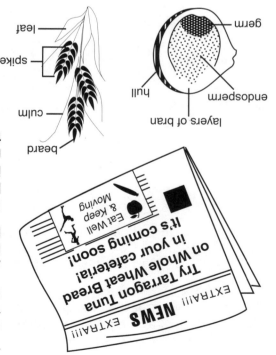

Whole Wheat Bread vs. White Bread

Try the wonderful world of whole wheat bread! It may look a little different, but whole wheat bread tastes good and is good for you. The more you eat it, the more you'll like it!

And it's more nutritious than white bread. White bread is made from wheat flour, which has had the bran and wheat germ removed from the grain.

Even when the white flour is "enriched" by adding back nutrients, only 4 nutrients are added. Compare it to whole wheat flour–the enriched white flour lacks much of the fiber and 18 other vitamins and minerals found in whole wheat flour.

Wheat…"Amber Waves of Grain"

Although wild wheat was not native to America, wheat seeds were brought here by Columbus and European immigrants, who planted them across the country. Are you familiar with the phrase "amber waves of grain" from our national hymn, "America the Beautiful"? It refers to wheat fields that spread far and wide and looked as large and impressive as an ocean.

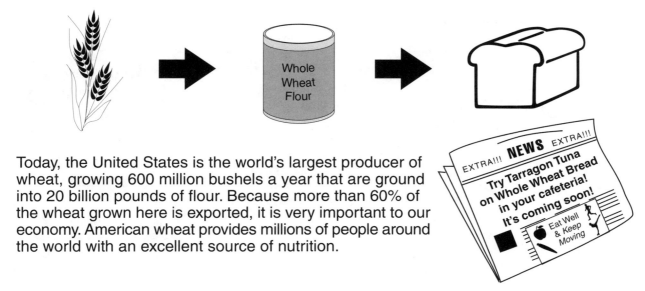

Today, the United States is the world's largest producer of wheat, growing 600 million bushels a year that are ground into 20 billion pounds of flour. Because more than 60% of the wheat grown here is exported, it is very important to our economy. American wheat provides millions of people around the world with an excellent source of nutrition.

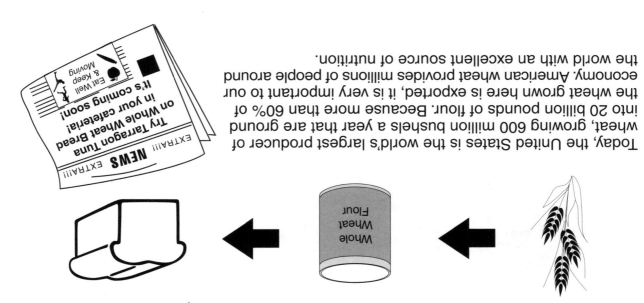

A Piece of the Pie?

Our days can be divided into many different parts. We sleep. We sit. We are active. The pie chart below shows how a lot of students, like you, spend their days.

How would your own pie chart look?

Sitting
11 1/2 hours

Being active
1 1/2 hours

Standing
2 1/4 hours

Sleeping
8 3/4 hours

The smallest piece of the pie is the "being active" slice. We all should try to make this piece much larger. Being active is important, and any kind of activity (walking, swimming, running) is better than no activity! So choose an activity to get those feet of yours moving!

Walk, dance, leap, hop, skip, jump, jog, skate, swim, run, and have fun!

Eat Well & *Keep Moving*

A Piece of the Pie?

Our days can be divided into many different parts. We sleep. We sit. We are active. The pie chart below shows how a lot of students, like you, spend their days.

How would your own pie chart look?

Sitting
11 1/2 hours

Being active
1 1/2 hours

Standing
2 1/4 hours

Sleeping
8 3/4 hours

The smallest piece of the pie is the "being active" slice. We all should try to make this piece much larger. Being active is important, and any kind of activity (walking, swimming, running) is better than no activity! So choose an activity to get those feet of yours moving!

Walk, dance, leap, hop, skip, jump, jog, skate, swim, run, and have fun!

Eat Well & *Keep Moving*

Be Wise…Warm Up for 5 Before You Exercise

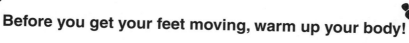

Before you get your feet moving, warm up your body!

Question: What is the very first thing you should do before you exercise?

Answer: Warm up for five minutes!

Five minutes = 1/12 of an hour: 300 seconds: 1/288 of a day

Why?

Just like warming up a car gets it ready to drive, warming up your body gets it ready for activity. Warming up also keeps you from getting hurt, which can happen if your muscles and joints haven't been loosened up.

How?

Do slow movements–like jogging in place or slow jumping jacks. Anything that keeps you moving slowly for five minutes will work!

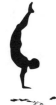 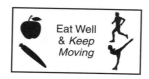

Eat Well & *Keep Moving*

  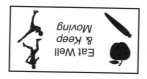

Question: What is the very first thing you should do before you exercise?

Answer: Warm up for five minutes!

Five minutes = 1/12 of an hour: 300 seconds: 1/288 of a day

Why?

Just like warming up a car gets it ready to drive, warming up your body gets it ready for activity. Warming up also keeps you from getting hurt, which can happen if your muscles and joints haven't been loosened up.

How?

Do slow movements–like jogging in place or slow jumping jacks. Anything that keeps you moving slowly for five minutes will work!

Before you get your feet moving, warm up your body!

Be Wise…Warm Up for 5 Before You Exercise

About the Authors

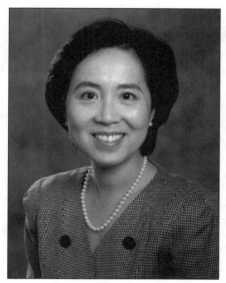

Lilian W.Y. Cheung, DSc, RD, is the director of health promotion and communication as well as a lecturer in nutrition at the Harvard School of Public Health, a respected nutritionist, and the coprincipal investigator who championed the creation of the Eat Well & *Keep Moving* program. The former director of the Harvard Nutrition and Fitness Project, Dr. Cheung coedited the book *Child Health Through Nutrition and Physical Activity*, which was among the first to recognize the importance of the dual role nutrition and physical activity play in children's health and disease prevention. She earned her master of science and doctorate degrees in nutrition from the Harvard School of Public Health.

Steven Gortmaker, PhD, is a senior lecturer at the Harvard School of Public Health. He is a widely known expert in children's nutrition and physical activity. He has appeared on national television and his work has been cited in the *New York Times, Wall Street Journal,* and other publications. Dr. Gortmaker was the coprincipal investigator of the Eat Well & *Keep Moving* program. He earned his PhD in sociology from the University of Wisconsin at Madison.

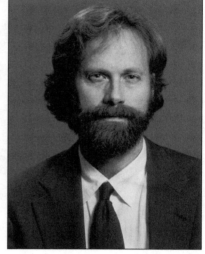

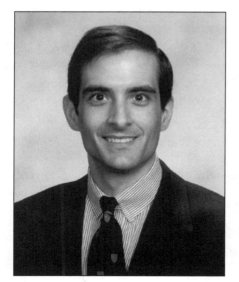

Hank Dart, MS, is a health communication consultant who works for the Harvard Center for Cancer Prevention, where he has helped develop the risk assessment/health education Web site, *Your Cancer Risk* (**www.yourcancerrisk.harvard.edu**). As manager of education and communications for the Eat Well & *Keep Moving* program, he directed the development of all educational materials. He has written many health-related guides and publications, conveying complex topics in easy-to-understand language for children and adults. He earned a master of science degree in health and social behavior from the Harvard School of Public Health.

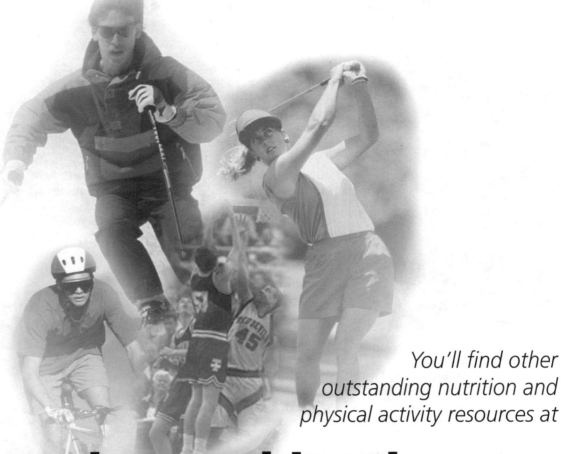